EMOTIONAL PROBLEMS IN LATER LIFE

Intervention Strategies for
Professional Caregivers

EMOTIONAL PROBLEMS IN LATER LIFE

Intervention Strategies for Professional Caregivers

DAN BLAZER

SPRINGER PUBLISHING COMPANY
New York

The six guidelines for managing patients given in Chapter 5 are abstracted from Morton, P. "Managing." *American Journal of Nursing* 25:28–33, 1987. Used with permission.

The mechanisms that may contribute to hypochondriasis listed in Chapter 7 are abstracted from Busse, E.W. "Somatiform and Psychosexual Disorders." In Busse, E.W., and D.G. Blazer. *Geriatric Psychiatry*. Washington, DC: American Psychiatric Press, 1989, pp. 429–458. Used with permission.

The guidelines for treating the hypochondriacal patient listed in Chapter 7 are abstracted from Busse, E.W. "The Treatment of Hypochondriasis." *Tri-State Medical Journal* 2:7, 1954. Used with permission.

The six personality types in Chapter 10 are abstracted from Kahana, R.J., and G.L. Bibring. "Personality Types in Medical Management." In Zinberg, E.N. (ed.), *Psychiatry in Medical Practice in a General Hospital*. New York: International Universities Press, 1964, pp. 103–123. Used with permission.

Some information in Chapter 12 is adapted from Chapters 2, 4, and 8 in Blazer, D., and I.C. Siegler. *A Family Approach to Health Care in the Elderly*. Menlo Park, CA: Addison-Wesley Co., 1984. Used with permission, Williams and Wilkins Co., Baltimore, MD.

The Chapter 12 discussion of roles that families take in working with older adults is adapted from Garetz, F.K. "Responses of Families to Health Problems in the Elderly." Paper presented at the 36th annual meeting of the American Geriatrics Society, April 1979. Used with permission.

The criteria for "wise judgment" outlined in Chapter 13 are adapted from Smith, J., A. Dixon, and P.B. Baltes. "Expertise and Right Planning: A New Research Approach to Investigating Aspects to Wisdom." Unpublished manuscript. Berlin, FRG: Max Planck Institute for Human Development and Education, 1985. Used with permission.

Library of Congress Cataloging-in-Publication Data

Blazer, Dan G. (Dan German), 1944–
    Emotional problems in later life : intervention strategies for
professional caregivers / Dan Blazer.
       p. cm.
    Includes bibliographical references.
    Includes index.
    ISBN 0-8261-7560-0
    1. Geriatric psychiatry. I. Title.
    [DNLM: 1. Affective Disorders—in old age. WM 171 B645e]
RC451.4.A5B56 1990
618.97'689—dc20
DNLM/DLC
for Library of Congress   90-8563
                                                                   CIP

Any medical or therapeutic agent or procedure described in this book should be applied by the practitioner under appropriate supervision in accordance with professional standards of care and the unique circumstances of each situation. Medically qualified readers are advised to consult the instructions and information included in package inserts of each drug or therapeutic agent before administration, particularly when using new or infrequently used drugs.

92 93 94 95 96 / 6 5 4 3 2

Preface

Professionals who work with older adults frequently encounter emotional suffering and/or dysfunction in these people. Coping with these emotional problems is a challenge to the elder, the family, and professionals serving them both.

This book is written to provide a better understanding of late-life emotional problems and strategies for professionals to use in overcoming those problems—especially those in health and social service occupations. I have focused on discrete problems of emotional functioning in late life, ranging from memory loss to anxiety, for problems are the usual trigger to "do something." Professionals are expected to act. What is to be done? The problem-oriented approach to the clinical care of elders suffering emotional problems as presented in this book provides not only a prescription for correcting those problems but a context for understanding their nature as well.

A problem-oriented approach to emotional problems is the foundation of sound clinical reasoning. It is through such reasoning that decisions for intervention are made and the comparative risks and benefits are weighed. For example, professionals working with older adults may encounter disruptive behavior in an elder who is suspicious. Effective investigation of the complaint uncovers the cause of the disruptive action and ensures an intervention that has the greatest probability of success. If the disruptive elder is acutely psychotic, a medication such as haloperidol (Haldol) is the most appropriate intervention. If the older person was placed in a strange environment, which precipitated the disruptive behavior, attempts at orientation and anxiety reduction are the most appropriate intervention. The outcome of the intervention trial is the only means by which a selected therapy can be evaluated for its effectiveness. Adjustments can then be made based on success or failure of the therapy, the preferences of the older person, as well as the economic and psychosocial costs (Goldman, 1987).

Problem-oriented clinical reasoning and decision making, however, can breed a sterility in work with older adults with emotional problems. A mechanistic approach to clinical care prevents professionals from knowing the older adult and the context from which the elder's problems derive. Henri Bergson, in his *Introduction to Metaphysics* (1961), describes the difference between intuition and systematic analyses. If we view 100 (or even 1,000) photographs of the city of Paris, taken from all possible points of view, we never derive the same experience as walking the streets of the city. In like manner, a complete "problem list" or even a complete biopsychosocial (and spiritual) evaluation of the elder can never be equated to the existential understanding of the older person obtained by dialogue and observation through time. Lab values, symptom lists, behavioral inventories, and functional assessments are no more than tools that enable professionals to rate observations and compare behavior across persons. The comparison across individuals comprises the science of clinical practice. The art of practice derives from work with each older adult within the context of his or her unique life experience.

I have taken a biopsychosocial approach to understanding the emotional problems from which older adults suffer. I describe the approach in the first chapter, and I have addressed the phenomenology, diagnosis, treatment, and management of each of the problems discussed in subsequent chapters from this holistic perspective. Regardless of the training of persons working with elders suffering emotional problems, each professional and caregiver must recognize the dynamic interplay of factors that contribute to the onset of problems, the persistence of problems, and the recovery from problems.

I have written this book from the perspective of a clinician and a clinical investigator. Not only do older adults with emotional problems present practical problems that call for intervention, they also express the range of feelings, behaviors, and their context during the later years. I have learned much about normal and successful aging by working with elders with emotional problems. I have learned much about emotional problems during the later years by talking with and listening to elderly friends and colleagues who appear to be aging successfully. I trust these insights will be of value to you, the reader.

I wish to thank the people who have been especially helpful in the preparation of this manuscript. First, Clyde Austin, Ph.D., and Bruce Davis, Ph.D., at Abilene Christian University emphasized the need for such a text and encouraged me to undertake the project. A. Jean Lesher at Scott, Foresman and Company was most helpful to me in formulating the approach and targeting the audience to whom I write. My son, Trey Blazer, typed the text and enjoyed pointing out inconsistencies and poorly written phrases. Denise Smith, my staff assistant, managed the logistics with skill and thoroughness, as usual. As always, my family—Sherrill, Tasha, and Trey—have been patient with the many weekend hours I spent in my study as I wrote this manuscript.

References

Bergson, H. *Introduction to Metaphysics*. New York: Philosophical Library, 1961.

Goldman, L. "Quantitative Aspects of Clinical Reasoning." In *Harrison's Principles of Internal Medicine* by E. Braunwald, K. J. Isselbacher, R. G. Petersdorf, J. D. Wilson, J. B. Martin, and A. S. Fauci, 5–6. New York: McGraw Hill, 1987.

Contents

CHAPTER ONE

Who Are the Elderly?

The number of persons 65 years of age and older will exceed thirty million within the United States by the year 1995, representing 12 percent of the U.S. population. As life expectancy increases and the baby boom generation ages, the number of persons over 65 will increase dramatically. Over fifty million persons who are 65 or older (21 percent of the U.S. population) are expected to be alive in the United States by the year 2020 (Atchley, 1985). The largest growing segment of the older population is the 85+ age group, over twenty times larger today than in 1900.

Most older persons are females and the advantage in life expectancy for females increases with age. The ratio of females to males over the age of 85 is greater than 2 to 1 (Atchley, 1985). Most older women are widows, for through much of this century, women married men who were older than they. The divorce rate among older persons has increased about four times in ten years between 1975 and 1985, though the rate of divorces in late life is less than 5 percent. Nearly half of older persons today have completed high school, compared to only one-quarter in 1970 (AARP/AOA, 1986).

In 1985, about 90 percent of older adults in the United States were Caucasian, 8 percent were black, and 2 percent were of other races, such as Native Americans or South Pacific islanders. Hispanics (a group comprising a number of races) make up about 3 percent of older adults in the United States (AARP/AOA, 1986). Blacks, Asians, and Hispanics are becoming an ever-increasing percentage of the older population.

Most older persons live in the community, and those in the community usually live in families. Eighty-two percent of older men and 57 percent of women live with family members. With increased age, however, the number of older persons living alone increases. About 5 percent of older adults live in institutions such as nursing homes or rest homes.

Despite the number of chronic illnesses suffered by older adults, most elders living in the community function with little or no impairment (Huntley et al., 1986). Over 95 percent of those in the 65 to 69 age range require no assistance in bathing, and over 70 percent in the 85 + age range can bathe independently. The same proportion by age can perform daily activities such as dressing (putting on a shirt, buttoning or zipping, or putting on shoes), walking across a small room, personal grooming (brushing one's hair, brushing one's teeth, or washing one's face), and getting out of bed and into a chair. When the requirements are more excessive, the percentages decrease. For example, over 70 percent of those in the 65 to 69 age group can perform heavy housework such as washing windows, walls, or floors, but less than 25 percent in the 85 + age group can perform these chores.

Older adults today are healthier and less likely to suffer economic hardship than elders earlier in this century. Nevertheless, chronic illnesses are frequent. Over one-half of older adults suffer arthritis, 42 percent suffer hypertension, 40 percent suffer hearing impairment, 34 percent suffer heart problems, 23 percent suffer visual impairment, and 8 percent suffer diabetes (U.S. Senate Special Committee on Aging, 1985; AARP/AOA, 1986). On the average, older persons' activities are restricted thirty-two days out of every year due to illness or injury. This number does not vary by gender. Elders accounted for 30 percent of all hospital stays and 41 percent of all hospital days of care in 1984 (AARP/AOA, 1986). Older adults are more likely to stay longer in the hospital, averaging nine days compared to less than six days for persons under the age of 65. They are also more likely to visit their doctor, averaging eight visits per year. Expenditures for their health care are greater than $120 billion per year, averaging nearly $4,000 a year for each person in 1985.

Out-of-pocket health care expenses for older adults are now about $1,000 a year.

Except for those suffering from dementing disorders, older adults are also less likely to be diagnosed as suffering from a psychiatric disorder if they are living in the community as compared to younger adults. For example, the prevalence of major or clinical depression is lower for the elderly (about 1 percent) than for any other age group (Myers et al., 1984). Yet many elders living in the community suffer clinically important symptoms of depression (8 percent in a study of elders living in North Carolina) (Blazer et al., 1987). Elders living in institutions are much more likely to suffer from psychiatric disorders (50 to 60 percent) when severe memory loss, secondary to the dementing illnesses, is included.

Successful Aging

Professionals working with older adults usually recognize problems with aging before they recognize successful aging. Research of aging has traditionally focused upon losses, such as loss of intelligence, loss of social roles, or loss of physical functioning. Clinical reports focus upon problems. If the elder, a professional, a family member, and society can prolong or eliminate the losses of aging, if a clinician can facilitate relief from or adaptation to the problems that the elder suffers, then we may falsely assume that aging is successful (Rowe and Kahn, 1987). Just as health is not the absence of illness, successful aging is not the absence of problems faced by the elderly. At virtually any age, we witness elders with minimal physiologic loss, elders who remain productive in society, and elders who are most satisfied with their lives. Successful aging is not easily defined, but each of us recognizes those elders who appear to age successfully.

A DEFINITION OF AGING

According to Busse (1989), *aging* can have several meanings. As a biologic term, it is used to describe those inherent biologic changes that take place through time and ultimately end with death.

By this definition, age would be the opposite of growth and development, those processes that begin with conception and end with the full maturity of an organism.

In practice, however, aging can be separated into primary aging (senescence), secondary aging (senility), and age-related diseases. Primary aging, a biologic process whose first cause is rooted in the heredity of the organism, produces an inevitable detrimental change that is time-related and independent of stress, trauma, or acquired disease. For example, bone loss increases in women at menopause, a hereditary biologic change within a woman. Secondary aging, in contrast, refers to defects and disabilities whose first cause comes from hostile factors in the environment, particularly trauma and disease. A calcium-poor diet and cigarette smoking are environmental stressors that contribute to secondary aging. Age-related diseases, such as osteoporosis, usually derive from both primary and secondary aging. By definition, the effects of secondary aging can be modified.

SOME CHARACTERISTICS OF SUCCESSFUL AGING

Although successful aging has yet to be fully defined; investigators usually agree upon the characteristics of successful aging. First, as emphasized by Rowe and Kahn (1987), *the results of aging must be separated from age-related yet modifiable risk factors for disease.* When, for example, the loss in bone density associated with aging (especially in women) becomes severe, the result is a fracture of the bones after a minimal trauma. Therefore, the age-related "disease"— osteoporosis—results in more than one million fractures in the United States each year. By the age of 65, nearly one-third of the women in this country have suffered a fracture of a vertebra, and by age 81, one-third of the women and one-sixth of the men have suffered a hip fracture (Riggs and Melton, 1986).

Are these fractures inevitable for the aging adult? No! There are factors other than age that modify the density of bone. One is the size of the individual. Persons who are heavier and therefore whose bones have been forced to carry more weight through the years are less likely to suffer osteoporosis. Carrying extra weight, however, is not the only way that loss in bone density can be prevented. Participation in exercise programs (such as daily walks) can slow the loss of bone density associated with aging. Calcium diet supplements appear to be of value in reducing bone loss in women. Other modifiable risk factors for bone loss include cigarette smoking and heavy alcohol intake. In other words, age is not the only determinant and may not be the most important determinant of bone loss, despite the relationship between increased age and decreased bone density.

A second concept necessary to understanding successful aging is the innate *heterogeneity* associated with aging. Maddox (1987) noted that professionals attempt to handle complexity by stereotyping (just as the lay public does). Scientists focus on central tendencies to capture the essence of a given process, such as the "classic case" of major depression, Alzheimer's disease, or myocardial infarction. Yet a report of central tendency when related to the thirty million persons in the United States who are 65 years of age or older does not inform us of the actual condition of a given elderly person. Are American elders poor, sick, depressed, dissatisfied with their lives, dysfunctional? Surely the answer is both yes and no; that is, the elderly cannot be described by central tendency and are best described by their heterogeneity. Even the average life expectancy worldwide varies from lows of 45 years in some underdeveloped countries to over 80 years in the more developed countries. Though most elders in the United States suffer at least one chronic medical problem, the majority do not suffer a disabling functional impairment. A recognition of heterogeneity encourages professionals working with older adults to plan their intervention to achieve optimal function rather than accepting the average functioning of older adults as a successful intervention. In actuality, few people are "average."

The Personality of Elders

Self-concept (or a sense of self) is the identity each person acquires, what each person thinks of himself or herself, how well a person believes that he or she has reached their potential, and how the individual perceives himself or herself integrating into the prevailing sociocultural environment. Yet "self," by its very nature, is a private matter.

Personality is the reflection of self to others. Personality encompasses our beliefs, habits, typical reactions to events (such as unexpected events), and our usual means of adapting to both rewards and crises in our environment. Our personalities develop throughout life with certain periods leading to greater changes than others. For example, adolescence is a time of considerable crisis in personality development. The early years of retirement also may be a period of accelerated personality change. The emotional problems experienced by older persons manifest themselves through changes in personality, such as introversion, as well as through simple complaints. Emotional problems place a strain upon the person, and adaptation to that strain may be an exaggeration of personality traits (see Chapter 10 for more information). To help a patient cope with his or her emotional problems, the professional must understand the patient.

What are the factors that contribute to personality? Most investigators now believe that heredity contributes much to personality. For example, the likelihood of similar personality styles (and even personality disorders) increases with identical twins when compared to fraternal twins. Anyone who has raised more than one child recognizes that the temperament of children varies and the differences in temperament, such as an angry temperament versus a fearful temperament, can be recognized early in the life of a child.

Cloninger (1987) reviewed the literature on the variants of personality and identified a consensus of three dimensions of personality: novelty seeking, harm avoidance, and reward dependence. Any given person may score high or low on those dimensions (Cloninger has developed a scale to measure persons along these personality dimensions—The Tridimensional Personality Questions [TDP]). Persons high in novelty seeking are impulsive, exploratory, excitable, and quick-tempered, whereas persons low on this dimension are reflective, rigid, stoic, and logical. Persons scoring high on the harm avoidance scale are cautious, apprehensive, fatigable, and inhibited, whereas persons who are low on the scale are confident, carefree, uninhibited, and energetic. Persons scoring high on the reward dependence scale are ambitious, moody, persistent, and sentimental, whereas persons who are low on the scale are self-willed, practical, tough-minded, and detached. Other dimensions can be constructed by combining two of the scales. For example, a person low on both novelty seeking and reward dependence is privacy-seeking, self-effacing, modest, and unimaginative. Cloninger takes his theory a step further by suggesting that these dimensions are genetically independent and are based on the excitation and inhibition of different chemical messengers, or neurotransmitters, in the brain. Novelty seeking is modulated by dopamine, harm avoidance by serotonin, and reward dependence by norepinephrine.

Costa et al. (1986) identified three personality dimensions (similar to Cloninger's): neuroticism (harm avoidance), extroversion (reward dependence), and openness to experience (novelty seeking). Their work is especially important, because they concentrated upon personality throughout the life cycle. Persons high on the neuroticism scale (though they may not suffer from a neurosis) tend to complain more about their health, are more likely to engage in health habits that are damaging (such as smoking and drinking), and are more likely to complain of sexual or financial problems. They tend to be more unhappy and dissatisfied with life and have a poor subjective sense of well-being.

According to Costa et al., extroverts prefer working in occupations where they have considerable contact with the public (such as social work or business administration). They enjoy being with others and have many social attachments, they tend to be more assertive and active, they tend to emit positive emotion, and they seek more stimulating experiences. Those who are more open to experience tend to engage more in fantasy and aesthetics, tend to rely more on their feelings rather than logic, are more spontaneous in their actions, tend to be free thinkers, and tend to have more traditional values.

Once basic personality style has been established (usually by early adulthood), these dispositions and traits tend to remain much the same throughout the life cycle. William James noted that, by the age of 30, the character is "set like plaster." Therefore, personality may contribute to adjustment problems in late life as older adults develop psychological and physical disorders. Personality traits, when exaggerated, can become maladaptive, leading to a so-called personality disorder (such as paranoid personality disorder, schizoid personality disorder, or antisocial personality disorder).

Personality contributes significantly to the presentation and the progression of emotional or physical problems arising in an older adult. For example, a man who tends to be suspicious and withdrawn will be even more reclusive and suspicious if his memory declines. The elder who is neurotic will exaggerate physical problems and subsequently have more difficulty adapting to physical disorders, leading to a decline in daily living activities and other functional capacities.

The Social Environment

Behavior, both normal and abnormal, also occurs within the context of family and society. Not only are most mental disorders caused in part by social factors, such as social stress and the lack of supportive social relationships, emotional problems and the resultant maladaptive behavior contribute to a disruption of the social environment. The social environment may be conceived from three different perspectives: discrete social stressors and chronic stressors, social support, and culture.

The first is the role of social stressors. Discrete stressful events can predispose persons to emotional problems later in life, precipitate emotional problems, or aggravate the course of an emotional problem. Losing a job in mid-life (even if a better job is found) may predispose a person to depressive symptoms and a sense of poor self-worth at the time of retirement. The loss of job at retirement is more difficult to accept as a natural transition and more likely to be interpreted as evidence of lack of competency. The loss of a loved one may precipitate a depressive disorder not unlike clinical depressions, although grief is not commonly considered clinical depression. If an elderly man loses his wife to cancer, his bereavement is difficult to distinguish from depression and may actually lead to a major depression.

If an elder develops an emotional problem in late life, the occurrence of stressful events during the course of that problem may prevent recovery. For example, a woman who becomes anxious following an automobile accident will have her anxiety aggravated by a close call on the road three weeks later. Stress, however, cannot be considered as solely a series of discrete events. Chronic stressors, such as economic hardship, the persistence of a chronic and potentially fatal illness, living alone, or conflictual family relationships may be more disabling than discrete stressful events.

Social stress is difficult to prevent. No one can guarantee that losses and hardships, such as an automobile accident or financial struggles, will not occur. Some factors in the environment, however, can modify the adverse consequences of both stressful events and chronic stress. Investigators who have studied these modulators of social stress perceive the social environment as supportive as well as stressful. Social support is the provision of meaningful, appropriate, and protective feedback from the social environment to the person that enables the person to negotiate intermittent or continual environmental stressors (Blazer, 1982). The concept of social support is attractive to mental health professionals, for it can be modified (improved), whereas many environmental stressors cannot be prevented.

The second aspect, social support, may be defined as follows:

- *Roles and available attachments:* The individuals and groups of individuals within the social network available to the older adult, such as spouse, children, and siblings
- *Frequency of social interactions:* The actual number of interactions within the social network; that is, how often an elder speaks in person with members of the social network or speaks with them by telephone
- *Perceived social support:* The subjective evaluation by the elder of his or her sense of a dependable social network, ease of interaction with the network, a sense of belonging to the network, and a sense of intimacy with network members
- *Instrumental support:* Concrete and observable services provided to the elder by the social network (such as food preparation, transportation, or nursing services) (Blazer, 1982)

The mechanisms by which social support buffer the individual from the challenge of a stressful environment are not fully understood. Cassell (1976) suggested that feedback, information, and guidance enable the older adult to understand and adapt to an ever-changing social network. These are the key factors.

The third aspect of the social environment of importance for understanding emotional problems in the elderly is culture. Aging takes place within a variety of cultures, and those cultures shape not only the aging process but the ideas of the society about aging as well. Culture provides the "context" within which life at a particular time and place occurs (Atchley, 1985). Culture is handed down from generation to generation and evolves gradually (although we experience occasional cultural upheavals). Culture exists mainly in ideas and their manifestations. These ideas, according to Atchley, include values, beliefs, norms, and stereotypes. *Values* suggest to us the relative desirability of certain goals. What is the most important goal for an older man, to maintain work or to relax and enjoy life? Many times, values conflict. For example, the need for financial security and self-respect, not to mention social recognition, encourages an elder to continue working. The desire for freedom from the problems of the workplace and the pursuit of pleasurable activities encourage early retirement. *Beliefs* tell us of the nature of the reality in which these values are based. According to Atchley, beliefs are assertions of what is accepted as true. *Stereotypes* are composites of more than one belief about a category of people, such as the widowed. Widows may be stereotyped as lonely, economically deprived, and not interested in relationships with persons of the opposite sex.

As culture changes through time, the historical period in which we live places a unique stamp on our values and beliefs. Most developmental psychologists affirm that the "formative years" are childhood through adolescence. Another formative period is the transition from adolescence to adulthood, usually occurring between the ages of 18 and 22. The nature of this transition is very much affected by the climate of the times in which it occurs (Atchley, 1985). For example, individuals who were born during the "roaring twenties" but sought their first work during the years of the Great Depression may have been forced to settle for work that was less than that for which they were qualified. Since 1945, however, the economic well-being for this birth cohort of older adults has steadily improved. Individuals born during the baby boom years (after 1945) may face a different economic stress, such as excessive competition during the years of their greatest productivity.

The year of birth shapes attitudes and values in late life and contributes to the prevalence and characteristics of the emotional problems of that birth cohort. For example, the cohort of older adults currently between the ages of 65 and 85 suffer a lower prevalence of clinical depression and suicide than the cohort that preceded them (over 85) and the cohort following them (45 to 65). Has this birth cohort been uniquely protected because they have experienced fewer physical, psychological, and social stressors during their lifetime than older cohorts? Evidence for a protective effect includes the increased life expectancy of this cohort (reflecting better health) and improved economic status compared to the birth cohort that preceded them in the twentieth century.

The Biopsychosocial Model

George Engel (1980), who recognized that the approach of professionals to their patients and clients is much influenced by the concepts around which their knowledge is organized, suggested a biopsychosocial model for the study and care of persons suffering physical and emotional problems. This model is especially applicable to the emotional problems that older persons experience and the context in which those problems occur. Engel used a common medical problem, a heart attack (myocardial infarction), as an example of the use of the model for understanding and coping with a problem.

Engel emphasized that nature is ordered hierarchically along a continuum, from complex larger units to less complex and simpler units. Each of these units interacts with other units. The units range from the biosphere through culture, community, and family to the person (the basic unit with whom most professionals work). Yet the person is a complex unit ranging from systems (such as the nervous system and the cardiovascular system) to tissues, cells, and molecules. Each system is composed of subsystems and each system is at the same time a component of a higher system. No aspect of the older adult suffering an emotional problem exists in isolation.

Clinicians and clinical investigators must select a level at which to concentrate, at least at the beginning of their inquiries and attempts to intervene, when they encounter an elder with an emotional problem. For most professionals working with older adults, the level addressed is the person—the client or patient served. Once a man suffering a heart attack contacts a professional and the problem is identified, the biopsychosocial model enables the professional to organize information regarding the onset of the event, the diagnostic workup, and intervention.

What happens during a heart attack? The artery, which supplies blood to the heart, is obstructed and this blockage leads to cell damage in the heart. When the cells are damaged, the heart can no longer function due to electrical instability and decreased ability to pump blood. The cardiovascular system adjusts to this blockage by feedback to the nervous system to activate emergency systems (such as an increased production of norepinephrine). The person experiences problems in the form of symptoms (which signal that the cells, tissues, and organ systems of the body are not working properly). These symptoms include pain and weakness and alert the individual to the emergency. The person then reacts in some way, such as seeking help from a family member.

The biopsychosocial model provides an excellent outline to understand a thorough evaluation. The health care professional encounters a person suffering the symptoms of a heart attack—sweating, severe chest pain, weakness, shortness of breath, and a host of emotional reactions ranging from denial of the problem to excessive fear and anxiety. The heart attack also exhibits itself at the cellular level, for the cell damage to the heart muscles deprived of oxygen increases the production of certain enzymes, such as AST (aspartate aminotransferase). At the tissue and organ system level, evidence of a blockage of the artery is found through the altered conductivity of electrical impulses through the heart. This change is reflected in the electrocardiogram (the principal diagnostic test for determining whether true damage to the heart has occurred).

Information from family members becomes most important, for if the older adult has complained of chest pain in the past, the nature and extent of the complaints at present must be distinguished from those of the past. Family members who identify the symptoms as being different and the behavior of the older adult as unique confirm a more serious medical event. Even at the societal level, impact on the diagnostic process is apparent. No chronic illness is more widely publicized in the United States than heart disease. More persons die of heart attacks than from any other disease. Therefore, the signs and symptoms of a heart attack are well publicized, which increases the likelihood that a person suffering a heart attack will seek medical attention as soon as possible.

From the perspective of treating the older adult suffering a heart attack, the biopsychosocial approach is equally applicable. If the victim resists and drugs are given that calm the heart and improve its efficiency during the initial recovery period, then tissue repair can progress at an optimal pace. Nitrates (nitroglycerin) increase the delivery of oxygen through those arteries of the heart that remain open and therefore improve the performance of the heart. Electrical stability of the heart is reestablished by a number of drugs (such as lidocaine) that calm the heart and reduce the likelihood of abnormal rhythms (which can cause sudden death). An increased oxygen concentration can be provided through the nose to reduce the strain on the heart as well.

At the level of the organ system, the organs of the body are allowed to function at a level requiring minimal blood flow through rest and close monitoring. Persons suffering a heart attack are admitted to a coronary care unit where they remain for three to five days under constant supervision with little activity permitted. They are fed a soft diet, which places decreased strain upon the gastrointestinal system, and they are provided with stool softeners, which decrease the strain of bowel movements. They are also sedated with antianxiety agents, such as diazepam (Valium), if needed. At this stage, some medications can be given that reduce the blockage of blood flow through the obstructed artery, such as heparin or streptokinase. Pain can be relieved by analgesics, including morphine.

The appropriate treatment of a heart attack, however, does not cease at the level of the cell or the organ systems. The person must be calmed and reassured regarding the nature and extent of the problem and the outlook for the future. Nursing staff on coronary care units have been trained extensively to provide such support to the heart attack victim. Though the immediate days following a heart attack are not the most appropriate time to engage in in-depth psychotherapy, professionals can address some acute problems effectively through supportive therapy and cognitive restructuring. The self-image of the victim, expectations and goals (which necessarily must change given the acute and severe illness), and the immediate fears must be addressed for effective treatment. Intervention does not cease with the patient. The victim must adjust relations with others, especially his or her spouse and children. Many heart attack victims were fiercely independent prior to the attack, and subsequently they must learn a more reciprocal relationship with family members, especially during the convalescent period. Nevertheless, the victim must not become too dependent in these relationships, thus disrupting the balance that has allowed the family to function prior to the heart attack.

Family members also require considerable support, for they must adjust to change in their valued elder, just as the elder must recognize a change in his physical capacities. Roles may be realigned and tasks may be redistributed within the family after the heart attack. Even adjustments within the community are required, for the older adult may have undertaken many community activities that now must be relinquished for the immediate future. Communities and cultures should evaluate their attitudes to individuals who survive a heart attack. Does a heart attack suggest that a victim invariably will be disabled or dependent? Education of the community can facilitate the receptivity by community members of the heart attack victim. Public health concerns about heart attacks even shape the governmental policies of health and delivery within state and national agencies. Massive efforts are currently under way to encourage persons of all ages to reduce their cholesterol levels by weight control, dietary changes, and exercise.

Professionals assist victims of emotional problems in a similar way to those helping heart attack victims. They use a model of intervention that encompasses the spectrum of the problem and employ interventions across the spectrum. As Engel cautions, the biopsychosocial perspective should not be construed as nonscientific. Though the model is more holistic and humanistic than the traditional biomedical model (one in which only the physical aspects of a problem are considered), data have emerged that enable professionals from any discipline to understand the emotional problems faced by older persons across the biopsychosocial spectrum. Emphases on different aspects of the model will vary from one condition to another. Hypochondriacal elders, by definition, suffer physical abnormalities that contribute little, if any, to their problems and therefore require greatest attention to the psychosocial aspects of the disorder. In contrast, when confronted with the dementing disorders, a thorough knowledge of the cellular, tissue, and organ system disruptions to the brain are as important as the psychosocial problems that accompany these disorders.

References

American Association of Retired Persons (AARP) and the Administration on Aging (AOA). *A Profile of Older Americans, 1985*. PF 3049 (1085). D996. Washington, DC, 1986.

Atchley, R. C. *Social Forces in Aging*. Belmont, CA: Wadsworth, 1985.

Blazer, D. G. *Depression in Late Life*. St. Louis: C. V. Mosby, 1982.

Blazer, D. G., D. C. Hughes, and L. K. George. "The epidemiology of depression in an elderly community population." *The Gerontologist*, 27:281, 1987.

Busse, E. W. "The myth, history, and science of aging." In E. W. Busse and D. G. Blazer (Eds.), *Geriatric Psychiatry*. Washington, DC: American Psychiatric Press, 1989. Pp. 3–34.

Cassell, J. "The contribution of the social environment to host resistance." *American Journal of Epidemiology*, 104:107, 1976.

Cloninger, C. R. "A systematic method for clinical description and classification of personality variance." *Archives of General Psychiatry*, 44:573, 1987.

Costa, P. T., R. R. McCrae, A. B. Zonderman, H. E. Barbarno, B. Lebowitz, and D. M. Larson. "Cross-sectional studies of personality in a national sample: 2. Stability in neuroticism, extroversion, and openness." *Psychology and Aging*, 1:144, 1986.

Engel, G. L. "The clinical application of the biopsychosocial model." *American Journal of Psychiatry*, 137:535, 1980.

Huntley, J. C., D. B. Brock, A. M. Ostfeld, J. O. Taylor, R. B. Wallace, and M. E. Lafferty. *Established Populations for Epidemiologic Studies of the Elderly: Resource Data Book*. Washington, DC: National Institute on Aging, NIH Publication 86–2443, 1986.

Maddox, G. L. "Aging and well-being." Boettner Lecture, Bryn Mawr, PA, 1987.

Myers, J. K., M. M. Weissman, C. E. Tischler, C. E. Holzer, P. J. Leaf, et al. "Six-month prevalence of psychiatric disorders in three communities." *Archives of General Psychiatry*, 41:959, 1984.

Riggs, B. L., and L. J. Melton. "Hip fracture in elderly males." *New England Journal of Medicine*, 314:1676, 1986.

Rowe, J. W., and R. L. Kahn. "Human aging: Usual and successful." *Science*, 237:143, 1987.

U.S. Senate Special Committee on Aging. *Developments on Aging: 1986*. Doc. 66-335. 1987.

Suggested Reading

Busse, E. W., and D. G. Blazer (Eds.). *Geriatric Psychiatry*. Washington, DC: American Psychiatric Press, 1989.

Zarit, S. H. *Aging and Mental Disorders: Psychological Approaches to Assessment and Treatment*. New York: Free Press, 1980.

CHAPTER TWO

Communicating with the Older Adult Suffering Emotional Problems

Author Norman Cousins, even prior to his report on his experience during a heart attack, recognized that physicians and writers had at least one thing in common—communication (Cousins, 1982). The ability to diagnose the problem presented to the clinician is a good test of that clinician's scientific competence. The ability to tell the patient what he or she must know is a good test of the art of medicine. Physicians and other professionals not only must be able to communicate effectively to older adults, they must hear accurately what the older adult is trying to say, even during times when the elder is reluctant to reveal the extent of a problem suffered.

The importance of successful communication is no more apparent than in facilitating older adults in coping with emotional problems. Even in this sophisticated age of diagnostic tests and biologic therapies, history taking and therapeutic communication remain the most important diagnostic and therapeutic tools available to the professional. The success of virtually any treatment depends on the adequacy of understanding the nature of the problem suffered by the older adult. The compliance of the elder with any approach to therapy (or even to a diagnostic test) depends on the professional's ability to understand the expectations and fears of the elder and to frame the advantages and disadvantages of diagnostic techniques in such a way that they can be comprehended (Blazer, 1978).

Communication is central to human behavior. The personality of the child is shaped through communication patterns between the child and parents initially, followed by teachers and schoolmates and later friends, family, and acquaintances in the workplace. When two persons are capable of communicating orderly and effectively with each other, adaptive behavior usually results from the endeavor. A disordered pattern of communication, however, can lead to emotional problems and maladaptive behavior (Ruesch, 1973). For example, an older adult who perceives the physician to be busy may believe that a medication prescribed is a means to "get her out of the office," is of no actual benefit, and may be harmful. The physician, on the other hand, once recognizing the multiple symptoms suffered by the patient as deriving from high blood pressure, sees no need to proceed further in the interview and prescribes a medication which he believes will be effective. At the extreme, many of the country's malpractice problems result more from poor communication between physicians and patients than from a lack of competence in medical care.

The following example illustrates the problems of communication between a professional and an older woman suffering from "nerves."

 Mrs. Freeman, a widow for three months, had deteriorated in her physical health to the point that she required a sitter for 18 hours a day. The family, concerned regarding her deterioration, sought consultation for her in a geriatric evaluation clinic. She was interviewed initially by a nurse to obtain background information. The interview progressed as follows:

NURSE: *Can you tell me why you are here today?*

MRS. FREEMAN: *My family brought me.*

NURSE: *I understand that you have not been feeling as well recently.*

MRS. FREEMAN: *I have been nervous.*

NURSE: *Can you tell me about your nerves?*

MRS. FREEMAN: *I have been nervous a long time.*

NURSE: *Do you think your nerves have become worse?*

MRS. FREEMAN: *I have trouble walking.*

NURSE: *But what about the nerves? Aren't you having difficulties since your husband died?*

MRS. FREEMAN: *My legs are swelling. Do you think support hose would help?*

NURSE: *Do you feel lonely at home since he has left?*

MRS. FREEMAN: *People stay at the house with me most of the time.*

NURSE: *It must be difficult having lost someone who you cared about for so many years.*

MRS. FREEMAN: *Can you do something about my nerves?*

NURSE: *Possibly you are nervous because you do not know what to do with the rest of your life, now that your husband has died.*

MRS. FREEMAN: *I do not think so.*

NURSE: *Is it that you just do not want to talk about the problems that you have?*

MRS. FREEMAN: *I am talking about my problems. My legs are swelling and I am having trouble walking. Can't you do something about this?*

NURSE: *We need to understand everything about you if we are going to help you.*

MRS. FREEMAN: *I am getting tired now.*

NURSE: *Can you tell me a little about your family?*

MRS. FREEMAN: *My daughter is outside. Why don't you talk to her?*

The interchange between the nurse and Mrs. Freeman should not be interpreted simply as a "denial" of bereavement. In fact, this conversation does not indicate whether Mrs. Freeman is actually suffering from the loss of her husband or not. Possibly, she had suffered a difficult marriage for many years. Possibly he had been ill during the latter years of his life. She may have even felt some relief at his death. The nurse also appeared to have difficulty in understanding what Mrs. Freeman meant when she complained of "nerves." Mrs. Freeman associated "nerves" with physical problems, such as the swelling in her legs and her lack of balance. She may have been concerned that the physical problems would progress and this was the reason she was "nervous." On the other hand, she may have viewed nerves themselves as being of physical origin and therefore requiring some attention. Mrs. Freeman apparently became frustrated that she could not make the nurse understand that she was troubled and wanted some help. She therefore, in disgust, referred the nurse to the family. The disordered communication between Mrs. Freeman and the nurse is not uncommon during the initial encounter between an older adult suffering emotional problems and a professional trying to help the elder. Many barriers limit therapeutic communication to evolve between professionals and elders. Some of these barriers are reviewed below.

Problems with Communication

PERCEPTUAL PROBLEMS

Disordered communication between professionals and older adults derives from a number of problems that span the biologic, the psychologic, and the social. A critical physical problem is sensory deprivation. As older persons have more difficulty in sensing and discriminating stimuli from the social environment due to a decline in function of the sensory organs, they have more difficulty in attending to and maintaining a conversation. Difficulty with hearing is the most common and perhaps the most disabling of the sensory losses in terms of verbal communication. The hearing loss that normally occurs in the older adult, presbycusis, is almost taken for granted among older persons. In most surveys of persons over the age of 65, the majority complained of at least some problem with hearing.

There are two types of hearing loss, loss resulting from a conduction problem (the passage of sound waves through the ear to the sense organ) and sensorineural. A major cause of a conduction deficit is otosclerosis. In this condition, the three bones of the ear that transform sound waves into vibrations of the ear drum—the malleus, the incus, and the stapes—become less mobile or frozen. Subsequently, sound cannot be transmitted into the inner ear.

A sensorineural problem common in late life is shrinkage and dysfunction of the sensory cells in the inner ear (the organ of Corti). This shrinkage leads to a decreased ability to hear high-pitched sounds and low-pitched sounds. Changes also occur in the auditory nerve, which makes speech discrimination more difficult as age increases. Although most hearing problems in the elderly are mild to moderate, they nevertheless create problems in social situations, especially when distracting sounds compete for attention or when the elder is distressed.

Visual problems also plague older adults. An early problem, almost always corrected through the use of lenses, is presbyopia, a solidification of the crystalline lens. The previously flexible lens (which can shift from focus on distant objects to focus on objects near the face) hardens in a fixed position that can focus well on objects at a distance, but no longer can focus upon near objects, such as printed matter within 12 to 18 inches of the eyes. The use of "reading glasses" corrects this problem easily.

More serious problems include glaucoma and cataracts. Glaucoma is common in the elderly and, unfortunately, can produce irreversible loss of vision before the older person is ever aware that the problem exists. Decreased vision secondary to glaucoma and cataracts often limits the ability of the elder to read and watch television, means by which the elder maintains contact with current events. Glaucoma is caused by a blockage of fluid flowing through the different compartments of the eye, which leads to increased pressure within the eyeball and damage of the optic nerve. As the disease progresses from the periphery of the visual fields to the center, the deficits may not be noticed before they become moderately severe, leading to a tunneling of the visual field. In addition, glaucoma causes little pain in the early stages. Fortunately, glaucoma can be easily identified through testing the pressure within the eyes (a test that all older persons should undergo at least every two or three years). By taking medications, glaucoma can be corrected, but once the damage to the optic nerve occurs, these losses cannot be reversed.

Cataracts are opacities in the lens that lead to a reduced transparency of the lens. Older adults suffering a cataract may initially see images doubled. As the condition progresses, they experience great difficulty in distinguishing small visual stimuli. Cataracts can be treated by removing the lens and then replacing it with an artificial lens implanted in the eye, wearing a contact lens, or wearing glasses with very thick lenses.

Problems also develop in the brain that affect communication. Some elders experience disease in the brain that interferes with their ability to understand sensory stimuli to which they are exposed (even though they receive them without difficulty). The older person may hear the words of another but cannot derive meaning from these words. He or she may also not be able to read the words on a piece of paper or recognize familiar objects. Persons suffering a stroke can develop dyslexia (inability to read), pure word deafness (inability to comprehend a word), and amnestic aphasia (inability to recall names of objects or parts of objects). Brain tumors, infections, and strokes can also lead to problems in forming words and ideas.

These difficulties with sensing and perceiving stimuli relevant to effective communication are further complicated by difficulties with speech. *Aphasia* is the term applied to problems that persons have in speech. As noted above, one type of aphasia is the inability to remember the word that represents an object, although the object is recognized and can even be described. For example, the elder may be able to describe the function of a typewriter without being able to recall the name *typewriter*. Other problems include agraphia (difficulty writing), apraxia (difficulty following directions), and dysarthrias (difficulty in forming words). An early sign of aphasia is a breakdown in syntax of sentences. For example, the older person, viewing a pastoral scene, says, "That's house. That's tree."

CHARACTERISTICS OF ELDERS THAT PREVENT EFFECTIVE COMMUNICATION

Another problem that interferes with communication between older adults and professionals is the innate cautiousness of elders. The elder who remains intellectually functioning rarely makes errors of commission but is likely to make errors of omission. When a professional is seeking information about a particular problem, the older person frequently omits details that are important in explaining the illness. The elder also takes a longer time to respond to inquiries. When a professional is compelled to hurry an interview with the elder, problems arise in obtaining the data necessary to accurately evaluate the emotional problems suffered by the elder.

Other problems that can interfere with communication are unrealistic expectations of the professional by the older adult (Blazer, 1978). The elder often bases the perception of a current professional on past experiences. As the style of medical care delivery has changed dramatically over the past twenty to thirty years, elders are often disappointed in the quality of care they receive, for in years past, quality of care was associated with time spent by the professional talking with the older adult. Technologic advances may have dramatically improved the ability of the physician to accurately and quickly recognize the cause of problems that previously went unnoticed. Nevertheless, the elder views the physician as uncaring when a treatment decision is perceived to have been made too hastily and is not carefully explained.

Older persons often perceive professionals as either parent or child surrogates. If the professional is viewed as a parent, the older adult tends to become more dependent in the relationship, frequently calling the professional for assistance, even to the point of daily contact. If the elder views the professional as a child, he may denigrate advice given by the professional and fail to follow instructions. Rather, the elder may lapse into providing instructions for the professional and even inquire into the health and behavior of the professional. Most often, older adults form positive, if distorted, views of professionals who work with them. These positive views (called positive transference by psychotherapists), when recognized, can benefit the professional in managing the elder.

THE PROBLEM OF "THEMES"

Another problem that obstructs effective communication between professionals and older adults is the problem of "themes." Physicians and other health care professionals focus on diseases. Older adults focus on their illness, that is, the pain and suffering they experience within the context of their lives at that time. Recognition of the characteristics of the "illness" is essential to effect communication with the older person suffering an emotional problem.

One theme is somatic concern. Elders spend much time complaining of ailments and may recount in exhausting detail problems with their physical functions (Blazer, 1978). When the older person is isolated or lonely, an illness can be not only a pain but also a blessing. Bodily problems distract the elder from sad remembrances of lost loved ones and isolation. In many ways, the elder's body keeps the elder company.

Another theme is the concentration on losses (Blazer, 1978). Elders usually adapt to losses, for loss is experienced frequently in late life. These losses include losses of friends, loved ones, employment, self esteem, role, and physical functioning (Blazer, 1978). The attitude of some elders toward aging is that the primary means to successful aging is to adapt to the progressive losses experienced.

A theme of great concern to older adults is losing control (Blazer, 1978). Fears range from the fear of losing control of bowel function to losing control over one's thoughts, in other words, "losing my mind." When the ability to regulate emotions decreases, the elder becomes ashamed and embarrassed. When the older adult can no longer drive and is dependent on others for transportation, the elder may fear social isolation.

Another theme related to illness in late life is the necessity of reviewing the meaning of one's life. Robert Butler (1963) has described the importance of allowing the older person to reflect and reminisce. The dissolution of function and dissociation from previous activities associated with approaching death stimulates the elder to integrate his or her past life. Integration is performed in large part by verbally reviewing the events of one's life, placing them in some order, and, through the organization of these events, finding meaning in life's experiences.

Still another theme is that older persons concentrate on death, often to the disturbance of both professionals and family members. Most elders do not fear death. Rather, their greatest fear is the fear of being alone at the end of life. As death is a topic not frequently discussed, the older person can be comforted if the professional honestly and openly discusses death with the elder.

SOCIAL BARRIERS TO EFFECTIVE COMMUNICATION

Barriers to effective communication do not originate solely from the older adult (Blazer, 1978). Attitudes toward elders by professionals ("old age means loss, incompetence, and constant physical complaining") can bias the professional in interacting with the older adult. Though Western society is aging, the emphasis remains upon youth. A middle-aged professional, attempting to maintain a youthful appearance through regular exercise, dieting, and attention toward physical appearance, often finds it difficult to empathize with the 83-year-old who appears somewhat disheveled, is no longer attractive physically, and whose physical agility has diminished. The professional working with an older adult must attend not only to the needs, concerns, and life view of the elder, he or she must also be aware of his or her own personal feelings about aging, the disabilities of aging, and even the meaning of life throughout life.

Attitudes, especially negative attitudes, toward older adults often emerge from a lack of understanding of the elder (Blazer, 1978). Professionals must separate myth from reality regarding aging. Older persons are labeled as senile, emotionally disturbed, unintelligent, or hypochondriacal. An unbiased understanding of normal aging and successful aging (see Chapter 13) will offset the negative attitudes toward older adults. In addition, the professional must put himself or herself in the older person's place and view life (perhaps a typical day) through the eyes of the older adult. What appears discouraging to the professional is frequently not discouraging to the elder. On the other hand, those problems most troublesome to the older adult may go unrecognized by the professional. Empathy is not easily taught in textbooks. Perhaps spending time with older family members or friends (not just a few minutes, but a few hours) will be of assistance to professionals in understanding the life of the older person. The middle-aged professional may be surprised at the ups and downs, the activities, and attitudes that are viewed within context of the actual living situation of the older person.

Techniques for Effectively Communicating with the Older Adult

AUGMENTATION OF SENSATION AND PERCEPTION

Whatever techniques can be used to improve discrimination of sensory input will facilitate therapeutic communication with the older adult. One of the most obvious (and yet most neglected) means to improve hearing is the use of a hearing aid. In the past, hearing aids have been viewed as suggestive of the impairments of aging because of their conspicuous nature; for example, the old ear horn used during the past century and cupping the hand behind the ear, a posture that reflects one of the more negative attitudes toward the elderly. The use of modern hearing aids is therefore viewed negatively by many elders. Yet electronic hearing aids can not only be effective in improving sensory input, they also are now shaped such that they are virtually unnoticeable. Stereophonic, that is bilateral, aids are much better than an aid for one ear. These electronic devices improve the threshold of hearing, increase the ability of the elder to discriminate speech, and assist the elder in determining the direction from which auditory stimuli derive (Busse, 1989).

Not all hearing loss, however, can be improved by the use of a hearing aid. In some types of deafness, the end organs (the hair cells of the cochlea) are virtually nonfunctional, yet the auditory nerve remains more or less intact. A single or possibly multiple-wire electrode can be planted in the cochlea to stimulate the nerve endings directly. This implant should not be confused with a hearing aid, for it does not amplify sound. Yet it does produce an auditory signal that can be learned and utilized by the severely hearing-impaired elder. Surgery can be performed to free the frozen small bones in the middle ear (the malleus, the incus, and the stapes) by replacing the stapes with an artificial metal or plastic device.

The improvement of visual reception to stimuli has already been discussed. Surgery, improved eyeglasses, and the use of contact lenses under certain circumstances can each improve the visual system of the older adult. Some visual problems with aging, however, cannot be corrected, such as senile macular degeneration and damage to the retina caused by diabetes. Careful control of diseases that make their onset in mid-life, such as diabetes and high blood pressure, can ensure improved vision in later life.

SPEECH THERAPY

Another approach to improving communication in the elderly is speech therapy. The older person suffering from aphasia and dysarthria can at times benefit from sessions with a speech therapist. These therapists are trained to assist the older adult in forming words, discriminating words (both heard and spoken) more effectively, much in the same way that a hearing-impaired child is trained in speech. Computer techniques that provide biofeedback regarding speech to the hearing-impaired child may be equally applicable in late life. When speech itself cannot be improved, elders can be taught sign language and lip reading. Television provides a useful source of training for lip reading. In addition, most metropolitan areas with cable television present a selection of programs that are translated for the hearing impaired through sign language (inserted into the screen). Sign language may be especially valuable to the emotionally disturbed hearing impaired elder who feels socially isolated. If the hearing-impaired older person has access to the electronic media, the perception of isolation may be decreased and the elder can then communicate intelligently with peers.

EFFECTIVE INTERVIEWING TECHNIQUES

The most important path to effective communication with the older adult suffering an emotional problem is the ability of a professional to conduct an effective interview with the elder. A number of techniques are of value for diagnostic and therapeutic communication (Blazer, 1978). The older adult should be approached with respect and dignity. If a professional is visiting the elder in a rest home or nursing home, he or she should knock on the door before entering the room, just as a physician should knock on the door before entering an examining room when a patient has come to the office. The elder should also be addressed by his or her proper names. Elders such as Dr. Jones, Ms. Ross, or Reverend Peterson, when they retire, are addressed as Johnny, Sally, or Jeff. These friendly and familiar references to older adults remind elders that their social roles have been redefined and they in turn are treated more like children than adults. At times, older persons give permission or even prefer to be called by their given names. Professionals, however, should wait for a cue that familiarity is permissible rather than assuming it is permissible because the elder is no longer in a professional role.

Health care professionals must be especially careful not to invade the privacy of the older person. Invasion of privacy is a common infraction occurring in hospitals and long-term care facilities. Few male physicians would enter the room of a 35-year-old woman until he was assured that she was properly robed. The natural inhibition to enter the room reflects the recognition of the sexuality of the patient by the physician. As the older adult may no longer be perceived as sexually attractive (or even sexual) to a younger health care professional, the inhibition declines and the physician bursts into a room when an elder is partially or even completely disrobed. The elder, however, is just as aware of his or her physical appearance and is as modest at the age of 85 as the age of 35. Assurance that the older person is properly robed must precede physical examination and, if disrobing is necessary, the professional should be accompanied by an attendant of the same sex as the elder.

During the interview of the older person, the professional should be positioned as near to the older adult as possible. Older adults are not nearly as reluctant to touch as younger persons and, because of difficulty with discriminating sensory stimuli, they appreciate a professional placing himself or herself as close as possible. The professional should be seated near enough to the elder to reach out and touch the elder if appropriate. The most comfortable arrangement of the chairs for both the elder and the professional is at a 45-degree angle to each other. The chairs should be of the same height and the professional should not stand or walk during the interview.

The professional should allow sufficient time for an interview with the older person. Time pressure has increased dramatically in recent years and medical technology has decreased the interaction time between physicians and patients. Yet the elder continues to view the interaction with the physician as a true "consultation," similar to the consultations of physicians and their patients during the nineteenth century. The consultative model of doctor-patient interaction was one such that the patient informed the doctor of everything that he or she believed relevant to the current problem (physical or emotional). The physician was skilled in asking those questions that "filled in the gaps" of the reported symptoms and often impressed upon the patient his or her thoroughness as a clinician by inquiring into areas that were later recognized by the elder to be of importance. Such consultations took time. There is no guarantee that professionals will have this time in the future, yet professionals working with elders should resist as much as possible the decreasing time allotted to professional/client interactions.

When I first evaluate an older adult suffering an emotional problem, I allocate 80 minutes, of which at least 50 are devoted to the elder and the additional 30 minutes to the family. Although persons with whom I consult are not wealthy, they rarely protest paying for the initial evaluation if they believe they have been understood by me and that I have a thorough understanding of the problems from which they suffer.

Next, the professional must speak clearly and slowly so the elder can understand. Even with proper lighting within the interview room (so that the elder can read the lips of the professional if he or she cannot hear) and the lack of distracting noises (so the elder can hear as clearly as possible), speech pattern contributes significantly to the ability of the elder to understand and respond to particular inquiries. The speech of the professional should be slow and clear. Simple sentences are the most effective means of communicating with the elderly, especially for those suffering hearing loss or memory loss. For example, only one question should be asked at a time, such as "How are you feeling today?" rather than "It is good to see you. How are you feeling today? It has been some time and I was wondering whether the sleep problems you complained of a couple of months ago have become worse." Clumping unrelated thoughts together inhibits the ability to communicate.

Older adults often communicate effectively by telephone interviews, for they can place the receiver of the phone next to the mastoid bone behind the ear and take advantage of bone conduction if they suffer mild to moderate hearing loss. Professionals should therefore not hesitate to use the telephone as a means of consulting with an older adult, at least for problems that do not require in-person evaluation. Telephone calls do not need to be prolonged, for they focus on a particular problem.

The professional must inquire actively and systematically into the emotional problems suffered by the elder. Older persons are reticent to reveal problems and may not recognize that the variety of symptoms they experience result from the same psychiatric disorder. For example, the depressed elder does not associate weight loss and sleep disturbance with the negative outlook on life and sense of hopelessness of the depressive disorder.

Systematic inquiry into emotional problems must be balanced with unstructured and undirected periods during the interview that permit the elder not only to state the nature of the problem in his or her own words, but also to connect both past and present. The onset of an emotional problem prompts the elder to review and reinterpret both present and past. Problems remind the elder of approaching death, decreased control over physical and mental abilities, and increased dependence on others.

The review, reminiscence, and apparent rambling of the elder can be frustrating to the busy professional who is attempting to acquire as much relevant data in as short a period of time as possible. Nevertheless, the professional must pace the interview in such a way that the older adult is given enough time to perceive that he or she has not only responded to inquiries by the professional, but also has related to the professional his or her view of the problem. Older persons, in contrast to many of us, are not uncomfortable in silences. Periods of silence provide an opportunity to think, formulate, and remember events and issues that are believed by the elder to be relevant to the current problem (Blazer, 1978).

ATTENTION TO NONVERBAL COMMUNICATION

To promote therapeutic communication between professionals and older adults, the professional must remain alert to nonverbal communication. Changes in facial expression, gestures, and even changes in posture suggest problems that are not apparent in the dialogue. For example, the depressed elder, though he or she does not complain of being depressed, may sit stooped over, appear sad, stare across the room, and avoid eye contact with the professional. During the interview, he or she is slow to respond and generates a message that the entire communication process is futile.

Touch is often an effective way to enable the older adult to relax, make better contact with the clinician, and to communicate more effectively. Older persons are less inhibited about physical touch than younger persons. If the elder senses a separation from the professional ("I feel out of touch"), then touch can bridge the communication gap, especially in the hospital or long-term care center. Holding a patient's hand or resting one's hand on the arm of the elder can be most reassuring and can improve verbal communication.

Honesty is an important element in any therapeutic communicative endeavor. Most older persons are realistic regarding the nature of their physical and emotional problems. If a professional makes light of a problem by saying, "There's nothing to worry about. You'll live to be a hundred," the elder will avoid the professional, thinking that the professional does not wish to understand the nature of the problem from which he or she suffers. As important as it is for the clinician to be realistic, it is equally important to remain hopeful. Hope can be generated by the professional if he or she concentrates on the here and now and avoids unrealistic expectations about the future. A few days free of pain are a great blessing to a terminally ill older adult but may be overlooked by the frustrated clinician who cannot cure the cancer.

As much as possible, professionals should make every attempt to continue relationships with older clients. Physicians especially should avoid transfers and terminations of the care of their older patients (Blazer, 1978). Older persons experience enough loss of persons of value to them. There are few reasons for terminating relationships with older persons, even if more specialized care is required. Health care professionals often become the most important persons to the older adult. The professional, therefore, must recognize his or her unique role in the life of the elder.

References

Blazer, D. G. "Techniques for communicating with the elderly patient." *Geriatrics*, 33:79, 1978.

Busse, E. W. "Perceptive changes with aging." In E. W. Busse and D. G. Blazer (Eds.), *Geriatric Psychiatry*. Washington, DC: American Psychiatric Press, 1989. Pp. 65–78.

Butler, R. N. "The life review: An interpretation of reminiscence in the aged." *Psychiatry*, 26:65, 1963.

Cousins, N. "The physician as communicator." *Journal of the American Medical Association*, 248:587 (1982).

Ruesch, J. *Therapeutic Communication*. New York: Norton, 1973.

Suggested Reading

Oyer, H. J., and E. J. Oyer (Eds.), *Aging and Communication*. Baltimore: University Park Press, 1976.

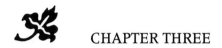

CHAPTER THREE

Memory Loss

Forgetfulness is among the most frequent complaints of older adults. Severe memory loss presents both elders and their families with the most challenging emotional problem and possibly the most challenging health problems in late life. Memory problems severe enough to cause social isolation and decreased abilities to function in family and society are not normal at any age. Nevertheless, two to three million persons in the United States suffer from primary degenerative dementia, a psychiatric disorder that leads to memory loss and a progressive decline in previously obtained intellectual functioning (Katzman, 1986).

The semantics of memory loss can be confusing. *Senility* is a term that has been taken out of context for years. The word actually means "degenerative changes associated with the aging process." Senile changes can occur in the eyes, the joints, and the kidneys as well as in the brain. *Dementia* is a loss of mental functioning that has previously been achieved during the normal development of the individual through the life cycle. Therefore, those persons who are mentally retarded—that is, they never achieved normal mental functioning—would incorrectly be labeled as "demented" in later life. *Senile dementia* (rarely used as a categorical term in recent years) was previously used interchangeably with *senility* to indicate the inevitable and appreciable loss of memory during the later years of life. *Senility* and *senile dementia* do not specifically indicate the nature or the cause of memory loss. Rather, they assume a type of "normal" memory loss that does not exist, and therefore should be abandoned as descriptions. Below is one example of an elder suffering loss of memory.

Mr. Jones, 77 years old and a successful farmer in North Carolina for most of his adult life, was asked by his family to consult with a psychiatrist because they were concerned that his judgment had deteriorated. He retired from active farming at age 67 and, after many years of intensive labor, enjoyed his rest and relaxation. Three sons and two tenant farmers continued growing tobacco, corn, and soybeans over his fertile 200 acres. He had negotiated an arrangement by which they would provide him a monthly portion of their income based on the success of the crop during the year. Never believing in banks, Mr. Jones received the payment in cash, as he had done most of his life, and kept it secured in his farmhouse.

Mr. Jones and his wife had few needs and therefore most of the income was saved. Neither his wife nor family became concerned about his banking habits until one day he could not account for much of the income accumulated over the past two years. The money had been secured somewhere in the twelve-room farmhouse (not in the usual hiding place) and Mr. Jones could not remember where he had put the money. About $25,000 had evidently been stuffed into books, dressers, cans, and other "banks."

On questioning, Mr. Jones was concerned that he had difficulty placing his hands on the money as quickly as he might like, but did not see this to be a major problem, as he continued to receive a regular income. Because he was increasingly distrustful of his sons, he was not inclined to tell them where he kept the money nor was he willing to let them care for his money. He believed his wife would give it to the sons and could not trust her with the money, either. Otherwise, Mr. Jones had no complaints. He slept well, ate well, and spent most of the day sitting on the porch or occasionally watching television. He expressed satisfaction with his life and little desire to do more than he was doing. Only with encouragement would he walk with his wife, yet did not feel any decrease in his energy.

During an examination of his mental functioning, Mr. Jones knew his name, that he had been brought to a doctor, and that it was the fall of the year (harvest time). He was confused, however, as to the year, the month, and the day of the month but did not feel that this was important, given that he no longer was forced to keep up with such things. He was given a screening examination in the office, the Mini-Mental State Examination, and he scored seventeen out of a possible thirty (see below for more information on this test). His score suggested borderline severe cognitive impairment.

Despite being disoriented, Mr. Jones denied any memory problems other than "what would be expected at my age." In fact, he was not aware that the family had encouraged him to seek this examination for memory difficulties. He believed his major problem was back pain, and he complained of this only occasionally. Throughout the interview, Mr. Jones was pleasant, showed neither symptoms of anxiety nor depression, and could follow questions without difficulty, although his answers tended to be brief and provided little information beyond what was asked.

Mr. Jones' doctor saw that he exhibited symptoms of senile dementia of the Alzheimer's type. He showed poor performance on an objective assessment of his cognitive functioning, the Mini-Mental State Examination. This exam is a thirty-item interviewer-administered scale that tests a number of cognitive functions, including memory, language skills, and motor skills. These functions become disrupted in the dementing disorders (Folstein et al., 1975).

His performance on the test, his family's recognition that he was not functioning as he once did (though they did not target memory problems as the reason for his dysfunction), his denial of memory difficulties, and his poor judgment all suggest a chronic and progressive dementia. Most old friends who talked to Mr. Jones would never have recognized his problems, however, for he had no disturbance in his consciousness and no difficulty in attending to a conversation. He had also learned, through short and noncommittal answers, to cover his memory difficulties.

Dementia of the Alzheimer's Type

Understanding the problem of memory loss is much like understanding a symphony. The theme or central movement is dementia of the Alzheimer's type. Yet there are many variations on this theme. The symphony of Alzheimer's disease represents the core symptoms of all of the dementias and can be contrasted with other dementing illnesses, such as multi-infarct dementia, alcoholic dementia, and Parkinson's dementia. The symptoms of delirium will then be described in more detail, followed by a discussion of diseases that tend to mimic dementia and delirium.

Dementia of the Alzheimer's type (DAT) is referred to as primary degenerative dementia, primary degenerative dementia of the Alzheimer's type, Alzheimer's disease, and senile dementia. It is the most common of the dementing disorders in western society. As many as 15 percent of those persons over the age of 65 may suffer at least early DAT and as many as 30 percent of persons over 80 years of age may be affected (Pfeffer et al., 1987). The likelihood of developing DAT increases dramatically with age, at least until the age of 85. If an elder survives to the age of 90, the likelihood of developing DAT does not increase, yet it does not decrease.

The cognitive (or thinking) problems experienced by persons suffering dementia span memory, language, attention, perception, and motor skills. The most pervasive problem is loss of memory. The DAT patient suffers disabling memory loss, especially of recent events. Family members are often surprised that a loved one can recall in some detail a vacation spent forty years ago, yet cannot recall having visited a son two days before. The older person does not appear to be that concerned about his or her memory loss.

Some memory loss does occur with advancing age. The average older adult "forgets, remembers that he forgets, and finally forgets that he forgets." For example, an older woman may forget the name of a new son-in-law. This memory loss troubles her, and she searches her memory until the name finally emerges. In contrast, the demented elder "forgets, forgets that she forgets, and could care less about her forgetfulness" after the early stages of dementia. The elder suffering from dementia, especially as the dementia progresses beyond the early stages, is more likely to cover or mask his or her memory loss than to express concern about it. Evasive answers or an expression of unconcern or frank denial (as exhibited by Mr. Jones) are prime examples.

LOSS OF COMMUNICATION SKILLS

Along with the memory loss, other problems accompany DAT. The demented person begins to lose the skill of communication. Specifically, the elder cannot complete long and complicated sentences and cannot recall words that are appropriate to a given conversation (aphasia). For example, the demented elder may have difficulty recalling the word "computer," although he or she can describe the function of the "machine that I type into which helps me to calculate my monthly budget."

LOSS OF ATTENTION

A third problem is loss of attention, though problems with attention generally do not emerge until late in the course of the disease. In contrast, attention is the primary problem experienced by the elder suffering delirium. For example, Mr. Jones could attend to the interview without difficulty, although another elder may become disturbed, fearful, and distracted.

PERCEPTUAL PROBLEMS

Late in the course of a dementia, the impairment to the brain becomes more diffuse. Problems in appropriately formulating what is seen and heard (perceptual problems) emerge. The older person can no longer read and understand simple messages or directives. For example, he or she, when asked to take a piece of paper, fold it in half, and place it in his or her lap, cannot remember the instructions and complete the task. Memory problems alone do not explain the inability to perform this task, for late in dementia the elder cannot assimilate the complex instructions.

DEPRESSION, AGITATION, SUSPICIOUSNESS, DELUSIONS AND HALLUCINATIONS

Early in the disease, moderate to severe depression is a common symptom (though many victims of Alzheimer's disease appear totally unconcerned). As the disease progresses, victims may become agitated, unable to sit still or cooperate with even the simplest task. Suspiciousness, delusions (false beliefs), and hallucinations (seeing things that are not there) may occur. It is not uncommon for patients with DAT to suspect that family members or caregivers wish to harm them or are stealing their property.

ANGRY OUTBURSTS

At times, the demented elder will lash out unexpectedly (especially when asked questions that are difficult to answer because of the memory loss), and he or she may even become physically abusive. This "catastrophic reaction" is short-lived, and the older person apologizes for the angry outburst a few moments after it occurs. An hour, a day, or a week later, the outburst will be repeated. (Agitation, suspiciousness, and hallucinations also accompany delirium). The delirious patient, however, is more likely to misinterpret actual visual stimuli (illusions) that he or she sees. For example, the clock on the wall may be interpreted as a face, spots on the floor might be seen as bugs, or a rope may become a snake.

OTHER PROBLEMS

Needless to say, other problems emerge that become apparent to the family and can be evaluated in the physician's office. The demented older adult has difficulty with simple calculations such as knowing the correct change to obtain from a dollar bill. He or she cannot react quickly or effectively while driving. The elder may use poor judgment, possibly hiding money that cannot be located later. His or her personality may even disintegrate. A proper older man, as he becomes progressively demented, may make sexual overtures to friends or even strangers.

THE PROGRESSION OF THE DISEASE

Dementia of the Alzheimer's type is a progressive illness that begins with the most innocuous of symptoms, such as forgetting where familiar objects have been placed or becoming temporarily disoriented while driving to a familiar location (Reisberg et al., 1984). As the disease progresses, co-workers may report that the victim is not working as well as previously. Lifetime interests such as reading or watching television decrease, probably because the demented elder has difficulty retaining material or following the theme. Social withdrawal, initially due to embarrassment and later to lack of interest, soon follows. (These early symptoms, however, are not exclusive to dementia, for they also are symptoms of major depression.) Although the victim may be pleasant during social interactions, his or her fund of knowledge decreases and poor judgment becomes an increasing problem. Often families are forced to assume financial responsibility.

During the later stages of dementia, the older person can no longer live independently. Concerns for safety may prompt the need for constant checking and later continual supervision. The demented elder will leave the bath water turned on, leave the stove turned on, and so forth. He or she may even wander away from home. In the coldest months of the winter, most large city newspapers report at least one demented older person who has wandered away, only to freeze to death. Incontinence, degeneration of speech, increasingly disturbed sleep, and eating difficulties emerge near the end of the disorder.

Multi-infarct Dementia

Alzheimer's disease is not the only dementia, though it is by far the most common. The second most common, often co-existing with DAT, is multi-infarct dementia. In this disorder, the dementia results from multiple small strokes throughout the brain. Although the symptoms are similar to those described for Alzheimer's disease, the course is not gradual, but stepwise, and the deficits tend to be "patchy." For example, agitation and depression may be severe, whereas memory loss is only minimal. Neurologic symptoms, such as increased deep tendon reflexes, weakness on one side of the body, and difficulty with balance and walking usually accompany multi-infarct dementia. High blood pressure, especially a protracted history of poorly controlled high blood pressure, is associated with multi-infarct dementia. Thus, the disease is more common among males and blacks, because these two groups tend to have more cases of high blood pressure.

Alcohol Amnestic Syndrome

Prolonged use of alcohol may also cause a dementia called the alcoholic amnestic syndrome. Alcohol used over time can lead to a deficiency of the vitamin thiamine, causing direct damage to the brain. Neurologic symptoms such as poor balance often accompany the memory problem. A combination of alcohol use and DAT complicates the course of both disorders. It is sometimes difficult to distinguish the exact cause. As the alcohol amnestic disorder can be arrested by a cessation of alcohol use, memory difficulties may not inevitably deteriorate as they would for true dementia.

Other Causes of Dementia

There are other causes of dementia, but most are infrequent. Dementia often accompanies Parkinson's disease but usually only after the victims have suffered from the tremor and rigid posture (the common symptoms of Parkinson's disease) for many years. Pick's disease is more common in Northern climates (such as Scotland and the Scandinavian countries). The victim of Pick's disease exhibits some blunting of emotion in contrast to the exaggerated emotions of multi-infarct dementia (Cummings and Benson, 1983). A rare but interesting disorder is Creutzfeldt-Jakob disease, found mostly in the Far East. This fatal dementia is caused by a slow-growing virus and can be transmitted from one person to another. That a disease which resembles DAT is caused by an infectious agent has led some investigators to suspect that Alzheimer's disease also may be caused by a virus.

Delirium

Delirium is characterized by acute episodes of confusion, clouding of consciousness, reduced ability to maintain attention to the external environment, and an inability to shift attention from one external stimulus to another. The major problem in delirium is not memory loss, although memory loss usually accompanies a delirium. In contrast to the dementias, delirium is caused by disease states or toxins from outside the brain (such as an acute physical illness or drug intoxication) and is usually alleviated when the disease is treated or the toxic agent is removed. Persons who suffer dementia and delirium are most different in the appearances of their problems, as is apparent in the following example of an older adult with delirium.

Mrs. Bishop was an 80-year-old woman, living alone, who fell while walking down the steps after church on Sunday morning. She fractured the upper bone in her left leg near its attachment to the pelvis (a femoral neck fracture). Following evaluation by an orthopedic surgeon, it was decided that the fracture was not severe enough to require surgery but could be treated with traction and immobility. She improved during the next few days and appeared to adjust to the hospital without difficulty, although she did require a sedative at night—flurazepam (Dalmane) 30mg—for five days after being hospitalized.

Bored in the hospital, Mrs. Bishop typically requested the Dalmane at 8 P.M. and immediately fell asleep. She would sleep well until 2 A.M., when she became agitated and frightened and did not know where she was. This happened four nights after she first took Dalmane. The nurses could not understand this dramatic change in her behavior. When their attempts to calm her failed, they called the intern who was on call. The doctor frightened her even more, for she perceived him to be "a man in a white coat coming to take me away." He gave her the tranquilizer haloperidol (Haldol) by injection, and after the second dose she went to sleep. She became agitated again the next morning, but the agitation lasted only thirty minutes or so, and she calmed down and seemed to do well during the day.

She had little memory of what had occurred during the previous night. The sleeping medication was discontinued. Although she had considerable difficulty sleeping during the next two or three nights, she improved dramatically and three days later, when she was discharged from the hospital, she was sleeping well and the fear and agitation had disappeared. Two weeks later, when she returned to see the orthopedic surgeon for an evaluation, she reported no problem with the confusion that she had experienced in the hospital.

Mrs. Bishop became delirious because of the inappropriate use of a sedative agent, Dalmane. That she was hospitalized (in a strange environment) and was suffering from a medical problem contributed to the delirium as well. Delirium is often more acute during the night, thus leading to the use of the word *sundowning* to describe the agitated and confused behavior observed by evening-shift nursing personnel in hospitals. As with most cases of delirium, when the source of the problem is eliminated, the delirium will cease.

In contrast to the gradual progression of dementia, delirium usually presents itself acutely, either with a mild severity that is often unnoticed by hospital personnel and family members or with a severity that leads to patients barricading the hospital room door owing to fears that emerge during the evening hours. If the cause of the delirium is identified early, then the delirium can be reversed. If the disease persists, however, permanent brain damage may ensue. For example, the acute problems associated with alcohol abuse are delirious (such as intoxication). If alcohol use persists, permanent problems may develop.

The causes of delirium are much more numerous than the causes of dementia. Virtually any systemic illness, such as acute or chronic infections, chronic lung disease, chronic heart disease, and endocrine disorders (diabetes and thyroid disease) may precipitate a delirium. In addition, alcohol or medications (especially tranquilizers and sleeping pills) may lead to a mild or even severe delirium. Poor nutrition and fluid intake (not uncommon in older adults who live alone) may also cause delirium.

Mimics of Delirium and Dementia

A number of emotional problems, discussed in other chapters in this book, may mimic delirium and dementia. Depression in older adults is often thought to manifest itself by reported memory loss, although the likelihood that a depression is the exclusive cause of a memory problem is small. The possibility must be pursued, for depression is usually reversible, whereas dementia is not. Sleep problems may lead to wandering and agitation at night and to decreased alertness during the day, which may mimic early DAT.

The Etiology of Memory Loss in Late Life

HEREDITY

At the molecular level, much interest has been devoted to the possibility that Alzheimer's disease is hereditary. For example, doctors who treat Alzheimer's patients discover families in which the majority of members reaching late life suffer the disorder. The disease often emerges before the age of 60 in such families; these families are rare, however. That DAT clusters in families suggests that a gene may be passed from one generation to another, at least in some families. Recent explorations have supported the possibility that this gene may be located on the 21st chromosome. A small portion of the chromosome may be replicated in the Alzheimer's patient (St. George-Hyslop et al., 1987). An additional duplication of this chromosome causes Down's syndrome. Young persons suffering mental retardation from Down's syndrome exhibit the same microscopic changes in the brain when they die (usually in their thirties and forties) as Alzheimer's victims exhibit when they die (usually in their seventies and eighties).

PLAQUES AND TANGLES

Two typical cellular changes occur in Alzheimer's disease, plaques and tangles. Plaques are a collection of bits and pieces of nerve cells and supportive tissues collected in a material called amyloid. It is not known why plaques develop, but one interesting theory suggests that the amyloid (a protein) attracts the growth of nerve endings into the plaque. This process eventually cannot support growth and the cells disintegrate (Whitson et al., 1989).

Tangles are filaments normally found within the nerve cells which become intertwined, causing the nerve cell to appear very dark when observed under the microscope after being stained with silver. These damaged nerve cells also contain an excessive concentration of aluminum, yet no conclusive evidence exists to suggest that exposure to aluminum in the environment (such as from soft drink cans) leads to an increased risk for DAT.

CHEMICAL IMBALANCES

A chemical imbalance has been discovered to exist in the brains of DAT victims. One of the chemical messengers, acetylcholine, appears to be decreased in concentration (Perry et al., 1978). While acetylcholine is important to memory, one must not assume that the "cause" of Alzheimer's disease is the reduction in this chemical messenger, for the reduction may be the result and not the cause. Correction of this imbalance may alleviate some of the symptoms of DAT but not the progression of the disease.

CHANGES AT THE CELLULAR LEVEL
FOR OTHER DEMENTIAS

Other dementias are accompanied by different changes at the cellular level. Multi-infarct dementia is associated with death of cells and even entire groups of cells supplied by small arteries that are blocked. These strokes (infarcts) produce the memory loss and other changes. The cellular abnormalities in multi-infarct dementia are quite different from those of Alzheimer's disease, though the symptoms are similar. Alcohol anmestic syndrome is caused by a deficiency of the vitamin thiamine and possibly a direct toxic effect of the alcohol on certain portions of the brain, especially the lower portions, such as the mammillary bodies. In delirium, cells are dysfunctional because they cannot operate effectively, probably because they are suffocating from a lack of oxygen or interference with their usual metabolism secondary to the disease or toxic agent (such as drug intoxication).

THE ORGAN SYSTEM

During the process of DAT, the brain becomes progressively more dysfunctional and the intricate connections and feedback mechanisms break down. As cells die, connections between different parts of the brain deteriorate. Those brain mechanisms necessary to maintain homeostasis in the body, such as temperature regulation and fluid regulation, cease to function. As memory decreases, the natural drive to feed oneself, keep oneself warm, and so forth also deteriorate. As the body requires an internal balance for survival, once this balance is disrupted by DAT, health declines. Late in the disease, the Alzheimer's patient is therefore more likely to suffer infectious diseases, dehydration, and malnutrition. Although a specific event occurs that is labeled the cause of death (such as kidney failure), many persons suffering Alzheimer's disease actually die from this organ disregulation, leading to a disruption of the body's homeostasis.

CLINICAL SYMPTOMS

Clinically, it is the reaction to memory loss that is most apparent. The memory-impaired individual may deny the memory loss, thus jeopardizing financial and business matters, or even the safety of a spouse. As the environment is less comprehended by the subject, suspiciousness increases. For example, DAT creates "holes" in the constant surveillance and orientation to the environment. These holes tend to be filled with imaginary material which in turn leads to a considerably altered view of one's surroundings. Inhibition also decreases with time. A most proper older woman known for her decorum and restraint may dress inappropriately (or even provocatively), or make overtly sexual comments to the embarrassment of the family. Depression may also result early in the course of the dementia, but as the disease progresses, depressive symptoms tend to decrease. If they persist, they tend to be short lived. Nevertheless, none of these factors appear to contribute appreciably to increased memory problems. Rather, they appear to result from the progressive deterioration of brain function.

SOCIAL AND FAMILY EXACERBATION OF PROBLEMS

Social and family problems do not contribute significantly to memory problems, though the memory difficulties present significant problems to family members. Some investigations suggest that isolation may increase memory difficulties, yet little direct evidence supports this theory. Abuse of older persons and neglect, however (especially neglect of nutrition and hygiene), will exacerbate memory problems. Vitamin B_{12} and folic acid deficiencies precipitate memory loss that is potentially treatable. Older persons who live alone and eat alone tend to neglect their food intake, as their taste perception decreases and they are limited in obtaining the necessary food stuffs for a balanced diet. Sensory deprivation resulting from social isolation and sensory impairment may be a contributing factor, yet current knowledge is circumstantial. For example, lack of sensory input can precipitate a retardation in brain development early in life. Even in later life, animals living in enriched environments have been found to exhibit at autopsy an increased number of neurons and connections between neurons.

CULTURAL RECOGNITION OF DEMENTIAS

Dementia occurs in all cultures but may be more recognized in some cultures than others (Mortimer, 1988). Studies of this hypothesis are most difficult to effect, however. Not only are most of the psychological tests used for identifying dementia culturally biased (and therefore not easily compared across cultures), but the number of older people in nonwestern cultures is often too limited. They also may be an especially hardy group of elders because of their ability to survive a harsh physical environment. In more primitive cultures, a demented older person can be cared for and socially integrated more easily, for the problems arising from dementia are not in such conflict with the culture. For example, the demented elder may not be confronted with social demands such as abstract conversation, managing business affairs, and following complicated directions to go from one place to another.

The Diagnostic Workup

The foundation of treating and managing memory loss is assessing the nature of the memory loss. A variety of professionals—including geriatricians, neurologists, psychiatrists, radiologists, pathologists, psychologists, nurses, and social workers—combine their efforts to understand the problem in each older adult suffering the condition. Appropriate therapy depends upon an accurate yet comprehensive diagnosis. Accurate diagnosis in turn is dependent upon the collection of accurate data from the cellular to the cultural context of the disorder.

ASSESSMENT AT THE CELLULAR LEVEL

At the cellular level, assessment includes both an evaluation of the genetic/hereditary contribution to the disorder and identification of cellular changes that may be helpful in identifying the neuropathology contributing to memory problems. Evaluation of hereditary factors involves two different approaches. If a genetic abnormality, such as a partial reduplication of the twenty-first chromosome, proves relatively frequent, then the division of chromosomes in cells actively dividing (such as in bone marrow or lymphoid tissue or cultures of cells that divide less frequently such as fibroblasts), can be examined during division (metaphase) to determine the presence of additional chromosome material. It is unlikely that such a simple technique will produce a diagnostic test for dementia, as it has not been demonstrated thus far. New techniques using recombinant DNA technology may be used in the future to probe for specific genetic abnormalities in Alzheimer's disease if such abnormalities are uncovered through our current research efforts.

When specific cellular abnormalities in DAT are better delineated, then the development of a diagnostic test to identify a person suffering Alzheimer's disease becomes possible. For example, the amyloid found in the senile plaques described above has been thought by some investigators to be unique to Alzheimer's disease. Remnants of the protein have been found in the spinal fluid of DAT victims but not age-matched controls. If this is true, then very sensitive assays of these substances could locate pathology at the cellular level. Thus far, no such test is available. Currently, the only possible means of diagnosing Alzheimer's disease at the cellular level is brain biopsy, in which a minute portion of brain tissue is extracted and examined under a microscope in order to determine the concentration of plaques and tangles. There are many ethical problems to using brain biopsy, and the value of the technique has not been demonstrated sufficient to even consider it a useful diagnostic procedure regardless of the ethics.

THE COURSE OF THE ILLNESS

The diagnostic assessment of DAT is most developed at the level of the clinical interview. A careful history from family members, usually from two generations, assists clinicians in determining the time of onset and the progression of the memory problem. Most victims of the dementias are brought by family members to the clinician's office (since the DAT victim tends to deny the problem). The family can also provide information that can eliminate other potential causes of memory loss. Families should be encouraged to bring all medications (to rule out drug intoxication) and to carefully review for the clinician a history of head trauma or medical illnesses suffered by the victim. Previous medical and psychiatric problems should also be related.

THE MENTAL STATUS EXAMINATION

Memory is assessed in the clinician's office by a mental status examination. In this test, patients are asked to remember who they are, where they are, when they are there, and why they are there (person, place, time, situation). Short-term memory can be evaluated by asking the victim to remember two or three objects (e.g., apple, chair) for three to four minutes. Retention and recall can be evaluated by saying a sentence or a series of numbers and asking the elder to repeat them. Calculation and attention can be tested by asking the person to subtract 7 from 100 and continuing to subtract from the answer received for six or seven calculations (serial sevens). If serial sevens are too difficult (perhaps for educational reasons) then the victim can be asked to subtract 3 from 20 or to perform a simple calculation, such as informing the clinician of the amount of change that should be received if a loaf of bread is bought at the grocery store for $1.75 and a five-dollar bill were given to the checker.

The loss of the ability to name objects, such as a pen or a watch, can be tested by asking the person to name objects held up to his or her face. A professional can best evaluate aphasia (the inability to remember names), however, by simply listening to the conversation of the demented elder. Even simple terms, such as typewriter, computer, or automobile, may escape recall, and the elder is then forced to describe the object that she or he cannot name. Additional tests of brain functioning include asking the victim to copy a drawing, rearrange a puzzle, or to interpret a proverb, a test of the ability to abstract. One of the better tests for identifying early dementia is to determine if the older adult can abstract or classify objects into a common category (such as recognizing that apples and bananas are both fruits). These simple procedures can be combined in a standardized format like the Mini-Mental State Examination (MMSE) (Folstein et al., 1975) and the Blessed Dementia Rating Scale (Blessed et al., 1968).

MORE DETAILED NEUROPSYCHOLOGICAL TESTING

More detailed neuropsychological testing assists with the assessment and is of special value in documenting the progression of cognitive decline. In some cases, selected memory impairment can only be identified by such sophisticated testing. Memory can be evaluated by the Wechsler Memory Scale; language by the Boston Naming Test; problem-solving by the Wisconsin Card Sorting Test; and attention by the Continuous-Performance Test. If these tests are repeated through time with patients suffering Alzheimer's disease, clinicians usually witness a progressive loss of recent memory followed by problems with language and finally visual perception.

LABORATORY AND OTHER
DIAGNOSTIC PROCEDURES

Laboratory workup is essential, and laboratory procedures include a complete blood count to screen for anemia; a test of blood chemistries to uncover possible dehydration or malnutrition; a test of thyroid function; an assay of vitamin levels, especially B_{12} and folic acid; a urinalysis to screen for the possibility of a urinary tract infection or dehydration; a chest x ray to screen for the possibility of severe lung disorders, which may lead to a lack of oxygen to the brain; and an electrocardiogram, which may identify rhythm problems that contribute to short-term loss of memory and loss of consciousness.

Direct imaging of the brain can be obtained through computed axial tomography (CAT scanning) and magnetic resonance imaging (MRI). Unlike x rays of the skull (which have been available for many years), these new imaging techniques permit viewing the brain directly (actually, the tissue of the brain). Although no specific findings on these tests identify Alzheimer's disease, the appearance of areas of the brain that have died (infarcted areas) solidifies the diagnosis of a multi-infarct dementia. Shrinkage (atrophy) of the cortex of the brain is associated with Alzheimer's disease. An electroencephalogram (EEG) is not of diagnostic use. The EEG is typically slowed in the patient suffering from delirium and therefore is a useful test for identifying this disorder. If information is not available about the use of medications, a toxic drug screen can provide information regarding the use of both prescription and illicit medications (if it is performed early in the diagnostic process).

PHYSICAL EXAMINATION

The physical examination should include a complete evaluation of the different organ systems, beginning with the nervous system. Tests should be thorough for both the sensory and motor systems (vision, hearing, gait, coordination, balance). The cardio-vascular system is evaluated by checking the blood pressure, listening to the heart, and listening to the lungs to determine if fluid has collected secondary to failure of the heart. The pulmonary system (respiratory system) is evaluated by listening to the chest and noting the color of the individual to determine if adequate oxygen is delivered to the other organs. The skin should be examined to see if sores or ulcers (which could be contributing to an infection) have developed because of poor hygiene.

PERSONALITY CHANGES

The perceptive clinician will pursue with the family changes in personality that are associated with the memory loss. Although the clinician may concentrate on the memory loss (recognizing that other changes in the behavior in the individual are a result of the memory problem), the personality change may be most distressing to the family. Qualities that have endeared the older adult to the family, such as a loving and thoughtful disposition, may change dramatically over time, as the older person becomes restless, easily upset, irritable, and self-centered. Other outgoing and independent elders may withdraw, become passive and dramatically dependent upon families.

EVALUATION OF THE ACTIVITIES OF DAILY LIVING

A careful evaluation of the activities of daily living is essential. Can the elder continue to work? Can she manage her money? Is it safe for him to drive alone? Can he cook and clean house? Does she smoke, and if so, does she become a hazard while smoking? As the problem of memory loss progresses, clinicians must probe for increased problems in daily care. Can the elder bathe, dress, comb his hair, brush his teeth? Are they able to get to the bathroom without soiling themselves? Can they eat meals? Do they have problems with falling? Though dementia is a disease of the brain, it affects the mind and especially the daily activities of the person.

EVALUATION OF THE FAMILY

At the level of the family, the evaluation is no less important. Over time, the function of the family in the care of the dementia patient is often the most critical aspect of care. Who is the primary caregiver? If the disease progresses, what arrangements can be made for caregiving? How does the family feel about the possibility of the demented elder moving to a retirement community, a rest home, or finally a nursing home? What are the behaviors that most trouble the family? Many families are repulsed by incontinence and the resultant care required to prevent soiling and ensure cleanliness. Other family members are more distressed at the possibility that the elder will wander from the home and therefore require constant supervision. Do caregivers receive help and support from outside the home? Are they in touch with sharing groups or support groups? Are they taking advantage of the available home care services and other services relevant to the treatment of the demented older adult? To what extent are finances a problem for family members?

CULTURAL VALUE AND DETERMINANTS OF CARE

At the cultural level, clinicians and professionals working with elders must remember that cultural values drive both formal and informal care for demented older adults. The recognition in the United States over the past fifteen years that Alzheimer's disease is not a natural accompaniment of aging but rather a disease has not only fueled research into the neuropathology of the disease, it has fueled a restructuring of finances to include funds for appropriate diagnostic workups through Medicare and private insurance. In addition, the financial burden of the disorder has led policy makers to seriously consider alternatives to care that are both humane and yet efficient. These policies are still in flux (as catastrophic health insurance remains to be worked out in detail). No one at present can project the cost (both financially and socially) to provide humane care for the victim of Alzheimer's disease. Professionals must therefore keep abreast of the changing policies and programs available in order to best counsel families and patients.

Urban Care. Regarding informal care, different subcultures care for their elders in different ways. Among urban, middle and working class families where both spouses work, the ability to care for a demented elder in the home is limited. The likelihood that one member of such a family will stop work in order to provide full-time care for the demented older adult is limited, especially if that person has teenage children and pressing financial responsibilities. This urban, middle-aged generation has been called "the generation between," facing challenges in caring for both their parents and their children. We may expect increased burdens upon them in the future.

Rural Care. In contrast, rural families have traditionally cared for demented elders within the home, and with financial and educational assistance, they may be capable of caring for a demented elder over much longer periods of time. A generational "contract" often is operational in such settings. Children view their parents caring for their grandparents and subsequently assume the responsibility to care for their parents in the future if dementia ensues.

Culture in Flux. Culture, however, is in flux and one can never assume, given a particular family background, that the family will follow the norm of their culture. Nevertheless, clinicians must avoid placing families into a procrustean bed requiring a particular set of services and support for the demented. Understanding the family and the culture from which the family derives enables the clinician to develop a personalized approach so that the demented elder may be cared for humanely and safely, while at the same time permitting the family to continue to function in other areas.

Treatment for Dementia and Delirium

The purpose and expectation of the basic research into the dementias today, especially DAT, is to find a means to reverse the progressive molecular cellular changes that underlie the memory loss associated with the dementias.

PHARMACOLOGIC THERAPY

A number of drugs have been proposed for many years to enhance memory. These drugs include dilators of blood vessels (such as papaverine), stimulants (such as nicotine or Ritalin), drugs hypothesized to improve memory by improving the oxygen delivery to cells (Hydergine), drugs thought to improve the organization of memory tracts within the brain (pirazetam), and even drugs thought to reverse the aging process (Gerovital H3). None of these drugs has been demonstrated to be especially superior in improving memory (though some, such as Hydergine, may have a role in the treatment of the early dementias).

In recent years, new compounds have emerged that may reverse at least some of the immediate chemical imbalance. Physostigmine is an anticholinesterase agent. That is, the drug reduces the concentration of the enzyme that breaks down the chemical messenger acetylcholine. The concentration of acetylcholine therefore increases. In some studies, physostigmine has been demonstrated effective, at least for a few weeks or months, in improving memory among patients with mild to moderate DAT. A second drug that has received much attention in recent years is tetrahydroaminoacridine (THA). Following a report from a small study suggesting that the drug facilitated dramatic improvement in Alzheimer's victims, a large cooperative study was implemented by the National Institutes of Health. Unfortunately, many persons who took the drugs (approximately 20 percent) developed liver function abnormalities. Now studies of THA are under way using lower doses, and no liver abnormalities have emerged. The experience with THA should be a lesson to us: We must not become too excited that drugs studied among a small number of people who have not been evaluated carefully for potential side effects will become a panacea. Most investigators today do not believe that THA will prove any more effective than the drugs presently available. There are no memory-enhancing drugs known to be effective and safe. Nevertheless, the search continues.

In the case of delirium, there is no need to search for an attention-enhancing or memory-enhancing drug. The problem is corrected by removing the agent that causes the brain cells to be intoxicated or suffocated. Aggressive treatment of infections, lung problems, and heart problems, and removal of drugs that may be intoxicating will reverse the cognitive problems.

At the organ system level, the use of medications is more effective. Low doses of antipsychotic medications, that is, those medications that are used most often to control agitation in severely ill psychotic patients, are effective in reducing agitation, improving sleep, even improving appetite. Nevertheless, these drugs are not without side effects. Drowsiness, unsteadiness, and tremors often result from the use of drugs such as haloperidol (Haldol) and thioridazine (Mellaril). These side effects include dry mouth, lowering of the blood pressure upon standing, and constipation. (A severe side effect, tardive dyskinesia, will be discussed in detail in Chapter 5.) Close attention to nutrition and hygiene (with frequent medical checkups) is also essential in caring for the demented older adult. Behavior problems often cease when elders sleep well, eat well, and do not suffer chronic illness.

DIETARY INTERVENTIONS

Other attempts to improve memory include dietary intervention, especially increasing vitamin intake or the use of proposed memory enhancers such as vitamin E or foodstuffs with high concentrations of acetylcholine or its precursors (such as lecithin). There is some rationale for the use of lecithin as a foodstuff: it has a high concentration of choline, the compound from which acetylcholine, the chemical messenger known to be of importance in enhancing memory, is derived. Most clinical trials in which lecithin has been studied have not proven the effectiveness of the precursor lecithin. (Other investigators have attempted to improve blood flow to the brain or at least oxygen delivery to the brain by placing persons in hyperbaric chambers. These attempts have been unsuccessful.)

REALITY ORIENTATION

Considerable debate has centered on a therapy available for many years, reality orientation. Reality orientation consists of explicit and repeated orientation of the cognitively impaired and withdrawn elder to the physical and social environment. The technique was introduced by Folsom many years ago. In reality orientation, Folsom emphasized the importance of continuing a verbal communication with the patient. The patient should be addressed by his or her proper name and each time a professional interacts with the patient, he should introduce himself. Information should be repeatedly provided as to where the patient is and what is to transpire. For example, if a male nurse enters the room of a demented elder in a long-term care facility, he might introduce himself, "Mr. Johnson, I'm your nurse today, Mr. Raskind. Isn't this a beautiful morning? Did you enjoy your breakfast of eggs and bacon? Now I'm going to help you remove your nightclothes and change into a shirt and pants. Please raise your arms so that I can help you take off your gown and put on the shirt." Such commands are most important when techniques that may invite suspicion, such as drawing blood or giving medications, are asked of the victim of Alzheimer's disease. Reality orientation is used not only in long-term care facilities, it can be taught to families who care for demented elders in the home.

Little evidence has emerged that the elder suffering from Alzheimer's disease will exhibit improved memory during reality orientation. Yet the daily activities of the demented elder may improve and less medication may be necessary for controlling agitation (unless conflicts arise around techniques). Family members who learn reality orientation can provide assistance to nursing home personnel during special times of the day with tasks such as bathing and feeding. Many sons and daughters will visit their fathers or mothers in nursing homes near mealtimes and help feed the parent. They will use reality orientation constantly over 30 to 45 minutes during the meal to encourage adequate food intake. Not only does reality orientation provide family members and professionals with a technique for improving interaction with demented elders, it enables the older person to be treated, even in the midst of severe impairment, with dignity.

PHYSICAL ACTIVITY

As demented elders exhibit decreasing ability to perform activities of daily living and are at increased risk for accidents, routines must be developed that ensure nutrition and physical fitness. Physical activity, such as walking, should be encouraged, and if walking is no longer possible, passive exercises in bed or chair should be encouraged. Alzheimer victims can participate in calisthenics if the directions are simple. Music and television are means by which the older person maintains some regular activity, even if he or she no longer can appreciate the genius of a composer or the theme of a television program. Older persons who have been life-long readers may continue to enjoy holding reading materials, possibly looking at pictures, and even reading despite an inability to retain information from the book or magazine.

Assistance to the demented elder in dressing becomes especially important. Demented elders often resist attempts by family members or staff to dress them and usually some bargaining must transpire between the elder and family or caregiver within long-term facilities. More complicated apparel, such as belts, suspenders, or ties, can be eliminated. Dentures may also be problematic, but caregivers must persist, or at least change the diet of the elder to accommodate loss of dentures.

Bowel and urine incontinence occurs late in the course of dementia, but may be especially disturbing to the demented elder. The use of a diaper to control urinary continence enables the older woman (who is more likely to be the victim) to maintain social activities she could not otherwise. Bowel incontinence can be treated to some extent by establishing regular visits to the toilet during the day (depending on the life-long bowel habits of the older adult). For example, taking the elder to the bathroom after breakfast may enable the demented elder to defecate, and thus bowel incontinence is avoided for the remainder of the day.

LONG-TERM CARE

At the level of society, the available support has improved dramatically over the last ten years. The burden of care for the demented elder (until transfer to a long-term facility, which usually occurs late in the course of a dementia) falls upon the family. The Alzheimer's Disease and Related Disorders Association (ADRDA) has developed chapters throughout the country in most large and medium-sized communities. These groups hold regular meetings, usually inviting an expert, perhaps a neurologist who can relay the most up-to-date information regarding treatments, or a social worker who has knowledge about the latest insurance programs available for long-term care. The most valuable aspect of the meetings, however, is the interaction between family members who are caring for Alzheimer's victims. Emotional support and practical suggestions are shared which not only demythologize the mysteries of the devastating illness but also break down the isolation that surrounds the overburdened caregiver. That other families are facing similar problems and have learned to cope with these problems is a major source of encouragement to a family that has only recently begun to face the problem of memory loss.

Through ADRDA (or other agencies and programs such as memory disorders clinics), families can be referred to public and private programs that are developing to support Alzheimer's patients within the home. These programs include training caregivers, respite care (that is, relief from the continual supervision of an Alzheimer's patient for perhaps a weekend or an evening), programs that inform regarding financial support, visiting nursing services, and homemaker services.

Long-term care counselors need to understand that one of the most difficult decisions families face is the "nursing home decision." Does the person suffering Alzheimer's disease require institutional care? At what point in the course of Alzheimer's disease is institutional care necessary? How do you counsel a person with a mother who has always protested she never wanted to be in a nursing home, and that person promised that he or she would never place the mother there? As Alzheimer's disease is rarely complicated by major physical problems (at least through the first few years of the disorder), most victims will experience memory problems and a decline in caring for themselves that will require institutionalization only during the last months of their lives. Yet end-stage Alzheimer's disease is most difficult to manage in the home. Rash and ill-advised promises must be rethought in the context of the safety of the Alzheimer's victim as well as the competing needs of other family members. Support from physicians, social workers, and fellow family members (through organizations such as ADRDA) assist families in making these difficult decisions. A consultation by the family with a social worker is most valuable in deciding what resources are available, how to begin searching for a nursing home, the problem of waiting lists, and confronting the guilt of placing a loved one in a long-term care facility. Informing family members that they can visit the older person frequently and that the demented elder may not realize after a period of time that he or she has been moved from the home can be of much comfort to the family.

Our society has directed much attention toward interventions for DAT. Our culture, which has generally equated normal aging with healthy aging, has been quick to recognize DAT and quick to search for ways in which the disease can be combatted. Unfortunately, the prevalence of DAT, its severity, and the lack of an immediate answer to the multitude of problems suffered by DAT patients suggest that our culture must be realistic as well as energetic in its approach to DAT. For example, millions of research dollars are being directed toward finding a "cure" for DAT (or at least the cause of the disease). Because of our refusal to accept the reality of the disorder, we often neglect the very areas where we might have the most impact, such as rehabilitation, family support, and the control of the secondary symptoms that render life most difficult for the patient and for others.

References

Blessed, G., B. E. Tomlinson, and M. Roth, "The association between quantitative measures of dementia and of senile change in the cerebral gray matter of elderly subjects." *British Journal of Psychiatry*, 114:796, 1968.

Cummings, J. L., and D. F. Benson. *Dementia: A Clinical Approach*. Boston: Butterworth Publishers, 1983.

Folstein, M. F., S. E. Folstein, and P. R. McHugh. "Mini-mental state: A practical method for grading the cognitive state of patients for the clinician." *Journal of Psychiatric Research*, 12:189, 1975.

Katzman, R. "Alzheimer's disease." *New England Journal of Medicine*, 314:964, 1986.

Mortimer, J. A. "Epidemiology of dementia—international comparisons." In J. A. Brody and G. L. Maddox (Eds.), *Epidemiology in Aging: An International Perspective*. New York: Springer, 1988. Pp. 159–164.

Perry, E. K., B. E. Tomlinson, G. Blessed, et al. "Correlation of cholinergic abnormalities with senile plaques and mental test scores in senile dementia." *British Medical Journal*, 2:1457, 1978.

Pfeffer, R., A. A. Afifiaa, and J. M. Chance. "Prevalence of Alzheimer's disease in a retirement community." *American Journal of Epidemiology*, 125:420, 1987.

Reisberg, B., S. Ferris, R. Anand, et al. "Clinical assessments of cognition in the aged." In C. A. Shamoian (Ed.), *Biology and Treatment of Dementia in the Elderly*. Washington, DC: American Psychiatric Press, 1984. Pp. 15–38.

St. George-Hyslop, P. H., R. E. Tanzi, R. J. Polinsky, et al. "The genetic defect causing familial Alzheimer's disease. Maps on chromosome 21." *Science*, 235:885, 1987.

Whitson, J. S., D. J. Selkoe, and C. W. Cotman. "Amyloid B protein enhances the survival of hippocampal neurons in vitro." *Science*, 243:1488, 1989.

Suggested Reading

Henig, R. M. *The Myth of Senility* (revised). Glenview, IL: Scott, Foresman and Company, 1988.

McKahnn, G., D. Drachman, M. Folstein, et al. "Clinical diagnosis of Alzheimer's disease." *Neurology*, 34:939, 1984.

Mace, N. L., and P. V. Rabins. *The Thirty-Six Hour Day*. Baltimore: The Johns Hopkins University Press, 1981.

Raskind, M. A. "Organic mental disorders." In E. W. Busse and D. G. Blazer (Eds.), *Geriatric Psychiatry*. Washington, DC: American Psychiatric Press, 1989. Pp. 313–368.

Reisberg, B. *Brain Failure: An Introduction to the Concept of Senility*. New York: Free Press, 1981.

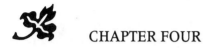

CHAPTER FOUR

Depression

"To be old is to be sad" is a theme that has persisted since antiquity. Simone de Beauvoir (1970), in the depressing book *The Coming of Age*, opens her discussion of the melancholy of later life with a description of Prince Siddhartha on one of his rides through the countryside. He observed an old, tottering, wrinkled, and graying man who was trembling, arthritic, and mumbling something incomprehensible even to himself. Turning to his charioteer, the young prince bemoaned, "It is the world's pity that we ignorant beings, drunk with the vanity of youth, do not behold old age. Let us hurry back to the palace. What is the use of pleasures in life, since I myself am the future dwelling place of old age?"

This view, however, was not universal. Esquirol, a student of Pinel, thought melancholy virtually absent in the aged. Older persons had lived "beyond the age of passion" and were therefore generally content and resigned. In addition, the nearness of death "inspired man with the desires of living." Esquirol mistakenly thought older persons are rarely suicidal. Actually, they commit suicide at a higher rate than any other age group.

In contrast to these poetic yet inaccurate views of depression and aging, recent research confirms that depressive symptoms are no more common in the elderly than in any other stage of life. Select groups of older persons may experience a higher prevalence of significant depressive symptoms, such as persons in long-term care facilities, persons suffering severe medical illnesses, or persons who are extremely isolated. Overall, however, life satisfaction among the elderly is as good (if not better) as any other age group. Life satisfaction is associated with good health, an adequate income, security, adequate social relations, and a sense of control over one's life. Though some elders may be at greater risk for losing some of the advantages, many (if not most) older adults are satisfied with their lives even into the last years of life.

Nevertheless, depression, especially the more severe depressions that require clinical attention, is among the more common and troublesome emotional problems facing the elderly. Among persons in the community, between 1 and 2 percent suffer a major or clinical depression. Dysthymic disorder, a more chronic and milder form of depression, is found among an additional 2 percent. Individuals suffering significant depressive symptoms secondary to adjustment (often adjustment to physical illness) make up an additional 4 to 8 percent. Among the medically ill and persons in long-term care facilities, clinical depression is found in about 12 to 16 percent, with an additional 20 to 30 percent suffering appreciable depressive symptoms.

Although the prevalence of major depression is lower among older adults when compared with persons in mid-life and early life, major depression remains an important problem to be faced by professionals working with older adults. The potential adverse results of depression, such as suicide, the neglect of health and hygiene, and the stress of depression on physical functions, underscore the necessity of recognizing the disorder and intervening appropriately.

THE MANY FACES OF DEPRESSION

Some years ago in a *Peanuts* cartoon, Charlie Brown was sitting at Lucy's psychiatric booth. He asked, "Can you cure loneliness?" She replied, "For a nickel I can cure anything." Charlie Brown then asked, "Can you cure deep down, black, bottom of the well, no hope, end of the world, what's the use loneliness?" Lucy protested, "For the same nickel?!" Both Lucy and Charlie Brown discover, upon exploring his problem in more depth, that depression has many faces. The many faces of depression in late life can be better understood by comparing the three depressed elders described below. Each suffers from a different problem.

Mrs. Sawyer, 70 years old and "without a care," complained to her family physician that she had lost much of her motivation and interest. The symptoms were not severe, yet she noticed that they had begun to interfere with her activities and dampened much of the pleasure she previously derived from her busy schedule. Her feelings were unexplained, though she believed, "I should feel better than ever," for many former family problems had been resolved, financial struggles had been overcome, and her good health continued. Though she loved her grandchildren, she found herself dreading their visit. Hobbies that she previously pursued had been discarded. At times she would stare into space for many minutes before she realized that her mind had wandered. An avid jogger, she had neglected her exercise program as well.

Mrs. Sawyer also reported difficulty sleeping. She awakened two or three times during the night and, for the last time, a couple of hours before her husband in the morning. Her appetite had decreased, and she had lost five pounds over three months. She perceived a decrease in her energy, though when forced to respond in a situation, she could manage her household responsibilities and social engagements. On occasions, she would find herself crying for no apparent reason. Yet what disturbed her the most was her loss of interest in virtually everything she did. Even when she accompanied her husband on a trip or was invited to a close friend's house for an evening meal, she had to force herself and found little pleasure from her efforts. These feelings were not acceptable to Mrs. Sawyer, for she had previously been a happy and secure woman.

Mrs. Sawyer's problem was that she suffered from a clinical depression, yet her symptoms were not severe. She never believed herself "emotionally disturbed" to the point that she would have sought psychiatric care. She was treated with an antidepressant medication, nortriptyline, and, almost immediately, her sleep improved and her crying spells ceased. Nevertheless, over the next two years, she never regained her motivation completely. The history of illness reported by Mrs. Sawyer and her response to medication is typical for many older adults. From the perspective of her doctor, she was successfully treated (for her sleep was better and she was functioning well). Nevertheless, the pervasive lack of interest continued to be troublesome to her.

 Mrs. Johnson was 70 years old when her husband died in April after a protracted illness. Her two daughters noticed, even at the funeral, that their mother was "not herself." Over the next month, she virtually stopped eating; she would only eat at the insistence of her daughters, who attended her throughout a meal. She would neither dress herself nor bathe herself, usually staying in her nightclothes during the day. She sat around most of the day staring into space and rarely spoke unless spoken to. When her daughters attempted to converse with her, she responded with irrelevant and "crazy-sounding" remarks. In May, she was taken to a neurologist, for her primary care physician believed her to be severely demented. Had she possibly suffered a stroke? Her daughters protested. She was doing well until the death of their father. "How could she lose her mind so quickly?"

When she was eventually evaluated by a psychiatrist, Mrs. Johnson said virtually nothing. The psychiatrist immediately suspected that she was suffering a severe, psychotic depression. He placed her in the hospital and started her on medications. Since she refused to eat, a nasogastric tube was placed into her stomach for feeding. Finally, the psychiatrist prescribed electroconvulsive therapy (ECT). After he discussed the necessity of the treatment and the expected outcome with both the patient and her family, all agreed to proceed with the treatments. Nine treatments later, Mrs. Johnson had returned to her former self. She left the hospital taking a low dose of lithium carbonate and was doing well three years after the hospitalization.

Mrs. Johnson suffered a severe, psychotic depression. Even medications were ineffective in treating her severe illness. ECT was successful, as it is for many older adults in reversing a severe depressive episode (see page 62 for further information). She suffered no recurrence of depression, and no further signs of "losing her mind" were noted by her or the family. Psychological testing six months later did not reveal any loss of memory. Some would diagnose Mrs. Johnson as suffering from pseudodementia, a "false dementia" caused by a severe depression.

 Mr. Paxton was 73 years old when he was hospitalized, once again, for shortness of breath and fatigue. He was seen by his primary care physician almost weekly because he suffered chest pains (secondary to

two previous heart attacks) and heart failure. A diuretic (water pill) and nitroglycerin alleviated the symptoms to some extent.

Mr. Paxton complained that he was just about ready to give up because he could no longer help around the house. Actually, there was no need for him to continue his former handiwork around the house, nor for him to attend to his large garden. His wife had assumed these responsibilities as he became more ill. Nevertheless, he felt useless and found himself spending many hours watching television. He was discouraged with the results of cardiac bypass surgery two years earlier following an acute heart attack, and he was frustrated that he was no longer the man that he once had been.

Mr. Paxton did not seek treatment for his depression, for he did not view his depression as abnormal or serious enough to require help. He became more animated when talking to his doctor, especially when he talked about his family and his many interests. He admitted he was watching too much television, yet he was an avid sports fan and he especially enjoyed basketball games. Visits from his children and grandchildren, who lived near him, were the highlight of the week, yet they did tend to tire him after an hour or so.

Mr. Paxton suffered an adjustment disorder with a depressed mood. He was having difficulty adjusting to a physical illness. The symptoms he reported are common among older adults who suffer chronic and severe medical illnesses. Antidepressant medications are of little benefit in treating adjustment disorders and actually may complicate the physical problem. That Mr. Paxton brightened when he became engaged in a conversation, even for a short time, suggested that he might feel less depressed if he could ventilate some of his frustrations regarding his illness. Psychotherapy could have been an effective treatment if he had wished to participate. He was not delusional regarding his illness, for he perceived accurately the nature of his problem and what he might expect over the months and years ahead.

THE VARIETIES OF DEPRESSION IN LATER LIFE

Depression presents itself in many varieties. The most important is *major depression* (clinical depression). In the current psychiatric nomenclature, the third edition of the *Diagnostic and Statistical Manual* (Revised) (1987), a person suffers a major depressive episode if he or she experiences a depressed mood and/or loss of interest or pleasure in one's usual activities. In addition, four of the following symptoms are necessary for the diagnosis: weight loss (or occasionally weight gain), insomnia or hypersomnia (increased sleep), agitation or retardation (a marked decrease in normal muscular activity), fatigue or loss of energy, feelings of worthlessness or guilt, difficulty concentrating (real or perceived), and recurrent thoughts of death or suicide. An elder may suffer a single episode of major depression, as did Mrs. Sawyer and Mrs. Johnson, or recurrent episodes.

Major depression is a serious condition and deserves the attention of a specialist. Even so, the severity of major depression varies significantly. For example, Mrs. Sawyer functioned relatively well, despite a depressed mood and four of the symptoms of major depression: sleep problems, difficulty concentrating, loss of interest in usual activities, and weight loss. Mrs. Johnson, in contrast, suffered a severe and incapacitating variety of major depression. Her illness was even life threatening.

Mrs. Sawyer, though she did not suffer a severe variety of depression, did suffer from a subtype called *melancholic depression.* Melancholic depression is characterized by at least five of the following: loss of interest (no motivation), lack of reactivity to pleasurable stimuli, symptoms worse in the morning, psychomotor agitation or retardation, significant weight loss, previous response to biologic therapies (such as ECT or antidepressant medications during an episode of depression), and a previous episode with similar symptoms that improved.

Mrs. Johnson suffered another variety of major depression, *psychotic depression,* which is characterized by delusions and/or hallucinations associated with severe dysfunction. Both melancholic depression and psychotic depression are thought to be more responsive to biologic treatments such as medications or ECT. Psychotic depression is relatively more common among the elderly compared to persons in mid-life. Older adults suffering psychotic depression usually respond well to ECT.

Recurrent episodes of major depression are sometimes interspersed with highs or manic episodes. *Manic episodes* are characterized by decreased sleep, excessive energy, expansive thought processes (which may result in the person taking on ill-advised responsibilities or making poor business decisions), an exaggerated sense of self and a loss of judgment. Through most of the life cycle, the mood of persons during manic episodes is expansive and euphoric, but among the elderly, an irritable mood with frequent outbursts of anger is typical. Bipolar mood disorder (manic depressive illness) may be somewhat less common in late life.

Dysthymic disorder (chronic depression or depressive neurosis) is more common among older persons than major depression. To receive a diagnosis of dysthymic disorder, the older adult must suffer from depression at least two years. Though less severe, depressive symptoms must have been present for the majority of the time during the two years. Dysthymic disorder and major depression often coexist, for persons who suffer chronic depression are much more likely to develop a major depression, thus leading to "double depression." This chronic depressive syndrome appears to derive more from psychological and psychosocial factors than major depression with either melancholic or psychotic features.

An *adjustment disorder with a depressed mood* is distinguished from the above disorders because the symptoms of depression are linked to a physical or environmental stressor. Mr. Paxton suffered an adjustment disorder secondary to physical illness—the most common stressor that leads to adjustment disorder among the elderly. Retirement, financial difficulties, difficulties adjusting to a new social role, marital problems, and a change of residence may also contribute to adjustment disorder. Adjustment disorders are, by definition, self-limited. Some stressors, however, may persist for months and even years (such as a chronic illness), and a depressed mood may accompany the stressor throughout. In general, persons throughout the life cycle adjust to stressors and develop adequate means of coping over time. If depressive symptoms persist beyond a few months after the stressor is removed, then another diagnosis, such as major depression or dysthymic disorder, must be considered.

Grieving, or *bereavement*, should not be considered a mood disorder, for the feelings of sadness following a loss are part of the universal human experience. A lack of interest in one's surroundings, loss of energy, difficulty sleeping, episodes of crying, sighing respirations, and poor concentration are usual rather than exceptional in the months following a loss. Although no specific length of the grieving process can be assumed for an older adult, the symptoms of bereavement often reach their zenith around six months following a loss. Symptoms may worsen for one or two weeks around the first year's anniversary of the loss, but the second year is usually marked by a reintegration into family and previous (or new) roles.

Organic mood disorder is still another variety of depression. In this disorder, a physical abnormality (such as an illness or drug intoxication) directly causes the depressive symptoms. (Organic mood disorder is discussed in more detail in Chapter 9.)

The Etiology of Late-Life Depression

By its very nature, depression as a phenomenon evokes a multidimensional explanation of that phenomenon. Certain physical agents, such as drugs and alcohol, are known to be depressants and not only do they depress consciousness, they can lead to symptoms of depression. Temperament can determine mood as well. We recognize the "optimist" and the "pessimist," that is, people who may experience the same event yet interpret the event differently. The proverbial optimist sees the glass half full and the pessimist sees the same glass half empty. Stressful life events (social factors) contribute to depression as well. Most would experience a depressed mood if a loved one was lost. The origin of the varieties of depressive disorders reflects different primary contributors, yet for most depressive disorders, the spectrum of causation is operant across the biopsychosocial model.

HEREDITY

Major depression, especially when alternating with manic depressive illness (bipolar disorder), is more likely to be found clustered in families than would be expected by chance. Therefore, many investigators in recent years have probed for an hereditary origin of major depression. For example, Janice Egland has studied the Amish population in Pennsylvania. As the Amish community tends to isolate itself from the remainder of society, they also tend to inbreed. The marriage of cousins among the Amish is common. Genetic abnormalities tend to express themselves more often in populations that are inbred if the gene causing the abnormality is found in the population. Dr. Egland and colleagues (1987) have found families among the Amish with a very high prevalence of both major depression (single episode and recurrent) and manic depressive illness. She has even gone so far as to suggest that the gene (or at least one of the genes) causing depression is found on the sixth chromosome.

Hereditary factors, however, are less likely to cause depression among the elderly, except in those cases where the older adult has suffered depression, possibly many episodes, throughout his or her life. The likelihood that a relative of an elderly patient suffering major depression will also suffer major depression is lower than for a patient in mid-life. Nevertheless, this finding must be scrutinized carefully. The best studies of an illness are performed when many members of the family can be evaluated directly. The parents of the older adult, the siblings, and even the children are often not available for direct evaluation due to death, illness, or geographic separation. The elder may have a poor memory of psychiatric problems among relatives as well. Yet the finding of less genetic contributions to major depression among the elderly who experience the onset of depression for the first time in late life is probably correct. Genetic abnormalities usually (though not always) express themselves earlier in life.

IMBALANCE OF CHEMICAL MESSENGERS

For years depression was thought in part to be due to a so-called chemical imbalance. The chemical messengers or neurotransmitters in the brain were hypothesized depleted, especially norepinephrine and serotonin. Many bits of indirect evidence support a chemical imbalance at the cellular level as a contributor (or at least a correlate) of severe major depression. For example, the drug reserpine, which is used for treating high blood pressure, leads to a depletion of the neurotransmitter norepinephrine. In some patients treated with reserpine, severe depression develops. Once the drug is removed, the depression disappears. Many of the antidepressant drugs increase the concentration of these chemical messengers within the gap between nerve cells in the brain (the synaptic cleft). Not all of the evidence, however, is consistent with a chemical imbalance. Most of the antidepressant drugs must be taken for two to four weeks before improvement is effected. The chemical balance, however, is corrected almost immediately, that is, the concentration of the chemical messengers is increased.

If the concentration of chemical messengers is not the specific factor that contributes to a depressed mood, then investigators are forced to look elsewhere. In recent years, attention has been focused upon the site where these chemical messengers attach to the postsynaptic neuron (the neuron that receives the impulse). These receptor sites are specific for given chemical messengers, and once the messengers attach to these receptors, a stimulus can be passed from one nerve cell to another. Could these receptors in some way be disregulated, thus leading to a depression? Investigators have found that these receptors are "down regulated" and the biologic therapies currently used in depression restore these receptors to their normal activity. ECT is at least as effective, if not more effective, in treating depression, yet no evidence suggests that ECT changes the concentration of the chemical messengers. ECT is now thought to "reset" the receptors of the chemical messengers.

Are there differences across the life cycle in the concentration of these chemical messengers or in the regulation of receptor sites? The concentration of both norepinephrine and serotonin are thought to decrease with age. Other investigators suggest that, among the depressed elderly, the number of receptors for chemical messengers may be lower in late life than for persons in mid-life. Yet these findings have not proven conclusive. The current data regarding chemical messengers and receptor sites across the life cycle reveal more similarities than differences.

DISRUPTION OF THE ORGANISM DURING PHYSICAL ILLNESS

At the level of the organ and organ system, many systems are disrupted because of illness and lead to severe depression. Whether the system changes within the organism result from the depressed mood itself, stress from the environment and/or a genetic abnormality is not always known. In some cases, however, the cause of depression is clear. A cancer of the pancreas, leading to general debilitation of the organism, may first become apparent through the emergence of symptoms of severe depression. Persons suffering a decrease in their thyroid hormone (hypothyroidism) may report to their doctors a decrease in energy, increased lethargy, depressed mood, lack of interest in their surroundings—the very symptoms that define a major depression. These physical illnesses increase in their frequency (among the elderly) and are often unrecognized.

DISREGULATION OF ENDOCRINE FUNCTION

Disruptions of other organ systems are commonly associated with more severe depressions, though they do not necessarily cause the depression. These system dysfunctions have received much attention in recent years. The endocrine system facilitates control of many body functions within an ever-changing internal and external environment. Unlike the nervous system, which quickly responds to sudden stimuli, the endocrine system, through the secretion of hormones into the bloodstream, provides a gradual adjustment to slowly developing external events. Chronic stress, such as the stress of an older person perceiving himself unsafe whenever he walks the city streets, leads to an increase in cortisol secretion. Cortisol facilitates the organism as it prepares to confront perceived danger by increasing the availability of sugar (glucose) in the bloodstream for more energy (among other functions). The concentration of cortisol in the bloodstream is carefully regulated, for prolonged elevation of cortisol can be dangerous. For example, synthetic cortisol (in the form of a steroid drug such as prednisone) is often given over a number of months to persons suffering severe arthritis. The drug is essential to prevent musculoskeletal disability, yet severe side effects, such as wasting of the bones and weight gain, develop with prolonged use.

The control of cortisol concentrations derives from a feedback mechanism that involves higher regions of the brain which, when they sense a lower concentration of cortisol secrete corticotropin releasing factor (CRF). This factor is transported to the pituitary gland (which resides at the base of the brain) and stimulates the release of adrenal corticotropic hormone (ACTH). ACTH enters the bloodstream, travels to the adrenal gland (which is located on top of the kidney) and stimulates the release of cortisol. In severe depression, this feedback mechanism is impaired, leading to an overall increase in the concentration of cortisol. This finding has stimulated some to suspect that depression derives in part as a response to chronic stress. The persistent increase in cortisol concentrations may contribute to the symptoms and signs of depression or it may only serve as an epiphenomenon of the depression.

Cortisol concentration increases with age (Rosenbaum et al., 1984). In elders over age 75, the regulation of cortisol concentration appears to be disrupted. Disregulation of cortisol concentration may render the older person more susceptible to the adverse consequences of cortisol. Clinical studies demonstrate that cortisol concentrations in the depressed elderly are higher than cortisol concentrations in depressed persons in mid-life. Since cortisol in high concentration can cause damage to the brain in certain animals, this disregulation of the hypothalamic-pituitary-adrenal (HPA) axis in both depression and aging deserves further study.

DISRUPTION OF THE SLEEP-WAKE CYCLE

Another system that is disrupted during depression is the sleep-wake cycle. We still do not understand much about the need for sleep nor the specific events that lead to sleep and wakefulness. Yet the profound changes in sleep with depression suggest a desynchronization of our regular sleep-wake cycle. Sleep can be studied with an electroencephalogram (brain waves, or EEG), studies of the movements of the eyes, and respiration. By combining these three measures, clinical investigators have identified five stages of sleep. Four of these stages (labeled stages 1 to 4) progress from the lightest sleep to the deepest sleep and are characterized by gradual slowing of the brain waves. The fifth stage is characterized by rapid movements of the eyes and associated with dreaming (and therefore called rapid eye movement [REM] or dream sleep). Adults cycle through these five stages throughout the night (4 to 5 cycles), experiencing the first episode of REM or dream sleep, on the average, about an hour and a half after the onset of sleep. Prior to the first episode of REM sleep, the elder progresses from stage 1, through stages 2 and 3, to stage 4, and then returns to stage 3 and stage 2. In the depressed, a total time of sleep is decreased, the number of awakenings are increased, the amount of deep (or stage 4) sleep is decreased. Perhaps the most striking finding among the depressed, however, is the change in REM sleep. The first episode of REM sleep among the more severely depressed often occurs much earlier in the sleep cycle (less than one hour from sleep onset).

The changes that occur during sleep in the depressed also occur with normal aging, but not to the same degree. Older persons generally sleep less than middle-aged persons (although the differences are not profound). They awaken more frequently during the night, spend less time in deep or stage four sleep, and usually experience the first episode of REM sleep earlier in the night. These changes cannot be assumed to place the elder at greater risk to depression. Nevertheless, a further disruption of sleep by a severe depression in an older adult leads to profound sleep problems. Sleep difficulties are among the most common and most severe symptoms experienced by depressed older adults.

MOURNING AND MELANCHOLIA

Popular and professional literature is replete with examples of distorted thinking processes during depression. The psychological changes during depression throughout the life cycle produce the characteristic symptoms of the depressive disorders. Do these changes cause depression? Are they simply a manifestation of underlying biologic abnormalities or a normal response to noxious environment?

Sigmund Freud believed the dynamics of depression were interwoven with the psychological reaction to loss of an important relationship. Melancholia resembles the mourning that results when something of value (whether it be a spouse or an ideal) is taken away. Melancholia differed from mourning, however, in that melancholia only occurred among persons who were "predisposed." The predisposed individual was emotionally attached to the lost object at an unconscious level and experienced unconscious feelings of anger toward that which was lost. As anger was turned upon self, melancholic symptoms emerged. The melancholic would cease interest in the outside world, no longer develop loving relationships, and decrease activity. Feelings of self-reproach and even an unrealistic expectation of being punished would dominate the melancholic. Freud used the term *melancholic* to distinguish a normal from an abnormal response to loss. Except for both being abnormal, the term is used in a totally different way in the *Diagnostic and Statistical Manual of Mental Disorders* (1987) used by psychiatrists.

INTEGRATION VS. DESPAIR

Eric Erikson hypothesized that depression would result when older adults believed they never accomplished anything of value during their lives. Older persons frequently look back on their lives to find meaning and themes in past events. Attempts are made to reconcile previous events with current psychological development. When this task is successful, the elder acquires a sense of integrity and purpose. In contrast, if the elder cannot find meaning in his or her life, despair, dread, and hopelessness emerge. Because elders cannot change the past, when an older adult has difficulty accepting mistakes, omissions, and lack of accomplishment, the realization that the die is cast can be most threatening.

COGNITIVE DISTORTIONS

Aaron Beck proposed a third psychological theory of depression—cognitive distortion. Cognitive distortion leads older adults to view their past, present, and future experiences as negative and idiosyncratic. If an unpleasant experience occurs, the older adult may perceive him- or herself as the cause of that experience by some defect in self. For example, if the grandchildren do not visit, it must be because the elderly woman is boring. If she is boring, she is worthless. When she wishes to obtain something or achieve something, then a flood of insurmountable obstacles overwhelms consciousness and assures her that these goals cannot be achieved. Frequently, when she attempts to interact socially with her children and grandchildren, she views the experience as defeating or damaging. If the local grocer attempts to help her find an item on the shelf, she interprets the help as further evidence of her lack of usefulness. Depression therefore becomes a never-ending and self-perpetuating cognitive style.

STRESSFUL LIFE EVENTS

A stressful social and family environment contributes to both the onset of depression and the persistence of depression through time. A supportive social environment can mediate life stressors and protect the older adult. The role of loss from the social network has been described above and recognized since antiquity. King David, in the biblical book of Samuel, suffered severe depressive symptoms upon the loss of his son Absalom. Recent studies, however, suggest that a stressful social and family environment may have less impact upon the onset and persistence of depression among the elderly than in earlier stages of the life cycle (George et al., 1989). Perhaps elders have gained perspective on those events around them and subsequently are not so influenced by social stressors. For example, the loss of a loved one has often been contemplated by older persons, as they see such losses occurring to their peers frequently. Most older women recognize that they will probably survive their husbands, for they have a longer life expectancy and, among the present cohort of elders, women are generally younger than their husbands. Therefore, she has thought about, if not talked about, life during widowhood. Certainly she will grieve the lost spouse, yet she will have rehearsed the grief. Such preparation, although it can never anticipate the complexities and varieties of being single again, does provide some buffer against the stress of such a loss.

CHRONIC SOCIAL STRESS

Chronic social stress may be more deleterious to the mental health of the older adult than stressful events. Chronic stress has been less studied, for it is difficult to identify and measure chronic stressors. The older person who fears walking to the grocery store each day because of the danger of being mugged, the older woman who serves as a caregiver for her demented husband, and the elderly man who finds himself each year under greater financial strain may develop a depressive disorder that neither they nor the clinician associate with the chronic stressor. Stressful events, both acute and chronic, also affect the physical health of the older person.

Once an episode of depression has begun, both acute and chronic stress may fuel the persistence of the depressive episode. The older adult recovers, only to lapse into depression again after a few weeks or months as the stressor that precipitated the episode emerges again from the environment. For those elders hospitalized during a depressive episode (or who may be moved to a more protected environment), a return to a stressful living situation may exacerbate a recurrence of the depressive episode.

CULTURAL FACTORS

Cultural factors contribute not only to the frequency of depression, but also to the nature of the symptoms reported by the older adult. Western society is a multicultural society, yet universal trends can be identified that have an impact on most persons living in a Western country. Cross-cultural studies are the most obvious means of examining cultural contributions to depression. Yet a more relevant approach to cultural differences in modern Western cultures is to examine successive cohorts in a similar environment.

Culture is changing progressively in our society. Each birth cohort through the twentieth century has experienced a different cultural milieu at different developmental stages. Persons born in 1900 experienced World War I in late adolescence, took advantage of the economic boom in their twenties, struggled with the economic depression in their thirties, and saw their children fight in World War II when this cohort was in their forties. Since World War II, the well-being of this birth cohort has gradually improved. The economy grew through the 1940s and 1950s. Medicare became available to these people in their sixties, and they were more likely than previous elderly cohorts in this century to have a pension other than Social Security.

In contrast, a cohort born at mid-century (1950) experienced the Vietnam War during their adolescence, experienced an economic recession in their twenties, and saw relative economic growth in their thirties. We as yet do not know what the sociocultural experience of the so-called baby boom cohort will be as they age, yet they have higher suicide rates in their twenties and thirties than our current elders had at the same age earlier in the century.

Data have emerged regarding the prevalence of depression across cohorts (Klerman et al., 1985). The earliest birth cohorts of the twentieth century have relatively low suicide rates compared to cohorts that preceded them and cohorts that follow them (Blazer et al., 1986). Since depression is the most frequent cause of suicide, we might assume that the current cohort of elders also has experienced less depression across the life cycle than younger cohorts. Cross-sectional estimates of the prevalence of depression demonstrates just that. The prevalence of depression is highest among the baby boom cohorts and lowest among current elders. One must not be too quick to impose these cultural factors on a given individual, for an 85-year-old person in the latter twentieth century may be suffering individual stressors that lead to a severe depression. Yet from the statistical perspective, the current cohort of elders has been relatively protected from the burden of depression. If history repeats itself, however, we may expect the prevalence of depression among older adults to increase as younger cohorts enter late life during the first half of the twenty-first century.

Birth cohort also effects the presentation of depressive symptoms. Older adults are less likely to spontaneously complain of depressive symptoms, though if probed regarding feelings of depression, they are as likely to respond positively that they are suffering the blues and blahs as persons who are younger. These same elders are less likely to report guilt.

The Diagnostic Workup

Although no molecular genetic marker has emerged to assist clinicians in diagnosing a severe major depression, an accurate family history of depression, suicide, and/or alcoholism can provide assistance in the diagnostic workup. In some families, multiple members of each generation suffer from manic depressive illness or a unipolar recurrent depression. One use of this information is to predict the course of depression. If an older woman suffers the onset of depression and has a brother who previously was diagnosed as suffering manic depressive illness, then the woman is more likely to eventually suffer a manic episode than another woman suffering a first-onset major depression. Another clinical use of this information is in prescribing treatments. For example, if the daughter of an elderly woman has suffered a severe depression in the past and has responded to a particular antidepressant, then an appropriate first choice of an antidepressant for the elderly woman would be the same antidepressant.

LABORATORY STUDIES

The hospital laboratory has become increasingly important in assisting clinicians to diagnose depression and differentiate the various types of depression. A number of tests assist clinicians in distinguishing the varieties of depression or assist them in selecting and evaluating the effect of certain treatments. The metabolites or breakdown products of the chemical messengers (neurotransmitters) can be assayed to determine concentration in both blood and urine. Some years ago, depressed persons who exhibited low concentrations of a metabolite of norepinephrine were thought to respond to a certain type of antidepressant (imipramine) and persons with normal concentrations of this same metabolite were thought to respond to another antidepressant (amitriptyline). Although this laboratory finding has not proven effective in selecting a specific antidepressant, it does provide an example of how a routine laboratory procedure could assist in the diagnosis and treatment selection of the more severe depressions. Measurement of the concentrations of various chemicals in the blood, cerebral spinal fluid, and urine are the most accessible windows to the neurochemistry of the brain of the depressed older adult.

A number of diagnostic tests assess the organ and organ systems of the depressed elder. One test is the dexamethasone suppression test (DST). This test enables a clinician to evaluate whether one hormone regulatory system, the hypothalamic-pituitary-adrenal-cortisol system, is in proper regulation. A synthetic hormone dexamethasone (which is not measured by chemical assays of blood but which is recognized by the brain as cortisol) is given to a depressed elder. Eighteen and twenty-four hours later, blood samples are obtained and assayed for the concentration of cortisol. If the concentration is lower than normal, then the system is working properly: the brain has recognized the artificial cortisol, dexamethasone, determines that the concentrations of cortisol are above normal in the system, and therefore decreases the supply of cortisol in the blood. If the feedback mechanism is not working, as it frequently does not work in depressed elders, then the cortisol levels will be normal or even elevated.

The DST is not diagnostic for depression (half the persons suffering severe clinical depression will respond as normals to the test). Nevertheless, a positive test suggests that some biologic treatment, such as a medication, is indicated. Perhaps the most valuable contribution of the test is in tracing progress from given therapies. If an older adult is suffering a severe and treatment resistant depression, ECT may be prescribed. An abnormal DST that reverts to normal during the course of the treatment is predictive of a good clinical response, even if the symptoms have not improved at the time of the test.

PHYSICAL EXAMINATION

Additional diagnostic tests of importance to evaluate the organ-organ system abnormalities in depression include a thorough physical examination, for many diseases—such as hypothyroidism and cancer—may cause depression. Medications should be reviewed carefully, for many drugs, such as propranolol (Inderal), a commonly used medication for high blood pressure, may cause depression. Nutrition and weight must be accurately evaluated. Almost every older adult who suffers a severe depression will suffer a noticeable weight loss, usually ranging between five and ten pounds. The evaluation of sleep abnormalities has been described above.

CLINICAL INTERVIEW

The clinical interview is the foundation to evaluating depression in older adults. Family members as well as the elderly patient should be interviewed. Current symptoms, the length of the current episode, the history of episodes of depression in the past, use of drugs and alcohol and previous response to treatment for depression are documented by combining data from both patient and family. The severity of depression is best evaluated by determining the degree to which the elder "suffers" from the depressive symptoms, the extent to which function has been disrupted, and the risk of suicide. Many rating scales are available that assist in documenting the nature and severity of the depressive symptoms. For example, the Center for Epidemiologic Studies Depression Scale (CES-D) and the Beck Depression Inventory (BDI) have each been demonstrated to be effective in assessing self-reported symptom severity. Objective assessment of the severity of depression can be determined by using clinician-administered scales, such as the Hamilton Depression Rating Scale (HDRS) and the Montgomery-Asberg Depression Rating Scale.

A number of diagnostic instruments are available to assess the distortion in thinking of depressed elders, such as the Dysfunctional Attitude Scale. In this scale, the older adult is assessed for degrees of distortion in his or her thinking.

Evaluation of the social environment and the family are best accomplished during the clinical interview. A family history of depression, evidence of chronic stress on the family (such as poverty), a determination of conflicts within the family (such as sibling rivalry between two children of the depressed elder), and the availability of ongoing social and instrumental support to the elder from the family are critical factors in placing the evaluation of the origins, nature, and treatment in context.

Cultural (that is, cohort) bias may suggest to the clinician that certain situations, such as crowded living conditions, are intolerable to the elder when in actuality the situation is well tolerated, if not preferred. Other situations which to clinicians appear acceptable may be intolerable to the older person. For example, an older person may be extremely depressed because a son is not willing to change jobs and move to the city where the elderly person resides in order to care for his father. To place such a burden on a child—especially a child who has an established job and family to support—would be unrealistic, if not selfish. Nevertheless, the father may have been more than willing years prior to make such a change in order to care for his parents.

Treatment for Late-Life Depression

The clinical treatment and management of an older person suffering depression includes three therapies that must be coordinated if the elder is to derive maximal benefit. Biologic therapy, psychotherapy, and family therapy complement each other to assure success.

PHARMACOLOGIC THERAPY

When the depression is more biologic, treatment at the cellular level can be effected by the use of medications. Antidepressant drugs should be prescribed when the older person suffers more severe melancholia and usually more severe symptoms. The trade names of these drugs are well known to professionals working with older adults: Elavil, Pamelor, Norpramin, Tofranil, and Sinequan. These antidepressant drugs are called tricyclic, because their chemical structure consists of three rings. Each of these antidepressant medications works primarily at the junction of one nerve cell to another (the synapse). They block reuptake of the chemical messengers that are excreted from the end of one nerve cell (by attaching to presynaptic receptor sites) and attached to the cell that receives the stimulus and continues to transmit the stimulus (post synaptic receptor sites). The blocking of reuptake leads to an increased concentration of the chemical messenger in the space between the nerve cells.

Antidepressants also appear to have an effect on the receptors themselves by restoring the sensitivity of the receptors to normality. The exact mechanism by which these medications relieve the melancholic depressions is not known. One of the mysteries regarding these medicines is that, if they work, it usually requires between two and four weeks before the effects are manifest. Antidepressant medications are not "uppers." If nondepressed elders take the medication, most experience only drowsiness. (Actually, a low dose of antidepressant medication is one of the safer means for treating sleep problems in older adults.)

Antidepressant drugs are not enjoyable drugs to take, though they are usually tolerable. Most create some drowsiness and therefore are usually taken at night. As depressed elders frequently experience difficulty with sleep, this side effect actually is beneficial. Dry mouth, constipation, transient blurring of vision and, rarely, confusion or memory problems are other side effects. For antidepressant drugs to be effective, they must be prescribed in an adequate dose.

Many physicians are not aware of the need for an adequate dose and therefore do not recognize the benefit of the medications because the older person does not respond to a very low dose. On the other hand, older persons do not require as high a dose as persons who are younger. Antidepressants are most effective when used by physicians who have experience with their use in older persons.

The tricyclic antidepressants are not the only drugs available. Because of their side effects and the lack of total success in reversing depressive symptoms (about 70 percent of persons with severe depression respond to antidepressants), pharmacologists and pharmaceutical companies continue to search for new drugs with fewer side effects and greater therapeutic effect. The search has led to the discovery of some interesting and unique drugs now used to treat older persons. Trazodone (Desyrel) is free of many of the side effects of the tricyclic antidepressants (such as the dry mouth and constipation), yet is very sedating and leaves a "hangover" which many older persons do not tolerate well. Fluoxetine (Prozac) has few side effects and is effective with some elders when tricyclic antidepressants are ineffective. Nevertheless, the drug is "activating" and can contribute to an uncomfortable agitation over time. Because of the potency of this drug, one dose can be given every other day. A group of drugs called the monoamine oxidase inhibitors (MAOIs) may be effective in treating depression associated with anxiety. These drugs, however, also lead to agitation. Certain foods, such as red wines and aged cheeses, cannot be eaten when the drugs are taken; the MAOIs interact with tyramine from these foods to elevate blood pressure.

ELECTROCONVULSIVE THERAPY

If these medications are ineffective, and the depression is severe, electroconvulsive therapy (ECT) is the treatment of choice. ECT has received much adverse publicity over the years, yet the treatment is now used frequently for severe depression in late life. If one surveys psychiatric units in large medical centers, approximately 50 percent of persons receiving ECT are over the age of 60. Some clinical investigators believe that older persons are less responsive to antidepressant medications than middle-aged adults but are as responsive to ECT. Treatments usually are given in the hospital and are safer than many of the antidepressant medications.

ECT is not without problems, however. Memory difficulties following ECT, which are usually of short duration, can be decreased by using unilateral treatments (that is, the seizure produced by the treatment is induced in the nondominant hemisphere of the brain—the hemisphere that is less associated with memory). An older person who complains of memory problems during a depression may not tolerate the added memory difficulties that arise during a course of ECT treatments. Other side effects of ECT that were frequent problems in the past, such as small compression fractures of the spinal column, have been virtually eliminated with modern techniques.

Six to ten treatments are usually required. In most cases, improvement is evident after one treatment. One or two additional treatments are prescribed after the improvement is noticed. No one, to date, understands why ECT is an effective treatment for severe melancholic and psychotic depressions. Most investigators hypothesize that ECT somehow resets those same receptor sites that are effected by antidepressant medications. ECT clearly does *not* shock a person out of a depression.

PSYCHOTHERAPY

Psychotherapeutic intervention should begin with education. Depression produces demoralization and devaluation. Such negative self-attributes prevent the older person from seeking and cooperating with treatment. Either elders believe that they have brought the depressive feelings upon themselves or they believe it will create too much of a burden for their families if they are treated. Depression should be described to the patient and family as a disease. The nature of depression should be explained during the initial evaluation visit. A number of books and pamphlets are available to help the older person understand depression. For example, the book *Feeling Good, the New Mood Therapy* by David Burns (1980) is an excellent introduction to the origins of depression and means by which negative attitudes can be changed. The National Institute of Mental Health has recently begun a Depression Awareness, Research, and Treatment program (D/ART) to promote an understanding by persons suffering depression as to the nature of the illness and the types of treatments available.

Cognitive psychotherapy has been demonstrated to be effective in treating depression in older adults. In addition to educating the elder regarding the nature of depression, the therapist encourages the elder to change those attitudes that facilitate depressive symptoms. The focus of cognitive therapy is the "here and now," in contrast to traditional psychotherapy, which searches the past for solutions to current problems. Cognitive therapy usually requires fifteen to twenty-five weekly sessions and is therefore better accepted by most elders than the traditional insight-oriented, long-term therapies.

In cognitive therapy, the older person is encouraged to recognize the interaction between thinking and feeling, that is, he feels what he thinks and he thinks the way he feels. It often is difficult to disentangle which comes first (and perhaps what comes first is not important). For example, a depression that is primarily biologic may precipitate the "feeling" of depression (lethargy, difficulty concentrating, sleep problems, lack of pleasure), which leads to negative thinking (I am a lazy person). On the other hand, constantly thinking that no one cares, that the elder is socially isolated, and that the future will only bring misery can lead to problems with sleep, a decrease in appetite, a lack of energy, and a loss of pleasure in most activities.

Aaron Beck (1979), the founder of cognitive therapy, suggests a number of means for overcoming these negative thoughts. First, the elder should talk back to the internalized critic. When a negative thought arises, such as "I'll never be of value to my children again," the thought is written on a piece of paper. Then the thought is rationally evaluated. Distortions in thought become apparent, such as "They sure seem to appreciate me keeping the children for a few days."

Older persons who are depressed frequently lapse into inactivity. They do not dress in the morning, sit in a chair for most of the day, and stare at the TV set without concentrating on the programs viewed. Such behavior is self-defeating, for it reinforces the belief that "I am of no use to anybody. I'm just lazy and can't do anything." Cognitive therapists therefore encourage the older person to make a daily activity schedule. The schedule must be realistic (for failure to complete activities on an overcrowded schedule reinforces the depression). Each day, if some activities can be completed, then positive reinforcement ensues. The older person who suffers depression must work to eat and sleep regularly, get out of the house, and visit friends and relatives (even if he or she prefers to remain at home). If finances permit, the elder should schedule a vacation for a week or two to break the depressive cycle. Vacations are also useful in educating the elder as to how many depressing thoughts are associated with routine activities at home.

Another approach to overcoming negative attitudes is the "life review," suggested by Robert Butler (1963) more than 25 years ago. Older persons often devalue their lives. If encouraged to write an autobiography and make an effort to find meaning from their lives, they may recover a more balanced view that counteracts the retrospective discouragement. Children and grandchildren value a living history of their elder family member as well. A review may include writing a poem or song, accumulating family photographs, or exploring the genealogy of the family. The current interest among young adults in the earlier part of this century (as seen by the increased interest in antiques and relics from the 1950s) has increased the status of the past lives of older adults.

FAMILY THERAPY

Most clinicians working with older depressed persons recognize that they cannot be treated in isolation. Older persons rarely come to a clinician's office alone but are accompanied by a family member. Although the depressed elder has difficulty in making decisions to seek treatment, they are willing to listen to family members and appease them by a visit to the clinician. The clinician therefore must make every effort to ally with family in order to ensure cooperation with the biopsychosocial treatment plan. Assistance from two generations, especially when the depressed elder has been difficult to manage by a spouse, is especially important. Older persons do not, as a rule, resist the clinician speaking with family members. Most therapists, in fact, will visit with family members each time the older person is seen for medication management and psychotherapy.

One example in which working with the family becomes paramount is the depressed elder at risk for suicide. Suicide cannot be totally prevented and, as noted earlier, suicide is more common among depressed older adults than at other stages of the life cycle. When the risk for suicide is recognized, some preventive measures can be effected. For example, medications should be taken from the older person and placed in the care of a family member. Guns can be removed from the house and the older person can be watched carefully (to prevent wandering). Clinicians must be careful, however, not to place too much responsibility upon the family. If serious risk for suicide is determined, the older person should be hospitalized and the clinician should make this decision, thus taking responsibility from the family and decreasing the conflict between the older person and family members during a depressive episode.

Family members also appreciate instructions as to how they can best communicate with a depressed elder. How do you respond to someone who constantly devalues himself and never sees anything positive in the future? Family members can be instructed to empathize with the older person, such as "I hear what you are saying and I understand." At the same time, family members should be cautioned that they cannot convince the older person that there is a reason to live in the midst of a depression. Rather, they should remind the elder that he or she is not seeing things accurately because of the depressive illness.

At times elders may express that they no longer wish to live, yet they refuse to seek medical or psychiatric attention. In such cases, family members should be encouraged to band together and insist on a proper evaluation. Often one family member is hesitant to go against the wishes of a beloved elder, even if the potential for self-destructive behavior is high. Rarely, however, does a psychiatric evaluation and treatment of a severely depressed elder interfere with the dignity of the elder over time. Instead, effective treatment often returns dignity to the older adult.

Family members can also benefit from behavioral techniques that assist in weaning the elder from being overly dependent on his or her family. A depressed elder, like a demented elder, may wish for constant attention from the family, whereas other depressed elders may wish to remain by themselves.

Depression is a chronic and frustrating problem for professionals who are helping others throughout the life cycle. Yet there are many appropriate interventions for assisting depressed older adults. The attitude toward depression, however, should be encouraging, since there are many effective ways of overcoming depression. British psychologist Sir Martin Roth is fond of saying that "Where there is depression, paradoxically there is hope."

References

American Psychological Association. *Diagnostic and Statistic Manual of Mental Disorders* (3d ed.). Washington, DC: American Psychological Association, 1987.

Beck, A. T., A. J. Rush, B. F. Shaw, et al. *Cognitive Therapy of Depression*. New York: Guilford Press, 1979.

Blazer, D. G., J. R. Bachar, and K. G. Manton. "Suicide in late life: Review and commentary." *Journal of the American Geriatrics Society*, 34:519, 1986.

Burns, D. *Feeling Good: The New Mood Therapy*. New York: The New American Library, 1980.

Butler, R. M. "The life review: An interpretation of reminiscence in the aged." *Psychiatry*, 26:65, 1963.

de Beauvoir, S. *The Coming of Age*. Paris: Editional Gallimard, 1970.

Egland, J. A., D. S. Gerhard, D. L. Pauls, et al. "Bipolar affective disorders linked to DNA markers on chromosome 11." *Nature*, 325:783, 1987.

George, L. K., D. G. Blazer, and D. C. Hughes. "Social support and the outcome of major depression." *British Journal of Psychiatry*, 154:478, 1989.

Klerman, G. L., P. W. Lavoir, and J. Rice. "Birth-cohort trends in rates of major depressive disorders among relatives with patients of affective disorders." *Archives of General Psychiatry*, 42:689, 1985.

Rosenbaum, A. H., A. F. Schatzberg, M. S. MacLaughlin, et al. "The DST in normal control subjects: A comparison of two assays and the effects of age." *American Journal of Psychiatry*, 141:1550, 1984.

Suggested Reading

Billig, N. *To Be Old and Sad: Understanding Depression in the Elderly*. Lexington, MA: Lexington Books, 1987.

Blazer, D. G. *Depression in Late Life*. St. Louis: C. V. Mosby, 1982.

Blazer, D. G. "Affective disorders in late life." In E. W. Busse and D. G. Blazer (Eds.), *Geriatric Psychiatry*. Washington, DC: American Psychiatric Press, 1989. Pp. 369–402.

Blazer, D. G. "Depression in the elderly." *New England Journal of Medicine*, 320:164, 1989.

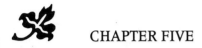

CHAPTER FIVE

Suspiciousness and Agitation

P*rofessionals working with older adults* frequently encounter suspicious or paranoid behavior often associated with agitation. Investigators who surveyed a community of elders in San Francisco found 17 percent to report that they were highly suspicious and 13 percent reported delusions. A similar study performed in North Carolina revealed 4 percent of older adults in the community experienced a sense of persecution by those around them (Christenson & Blazer, 1984). Ideas of persecution or perceptions of a hostile social environment increase stress and agitation among elders and thus render these elders among the more difficult with whom to work.

Of the suspicious or paranoid elders, a unique group has been recognized in Europe for years. This "late life paraphrenia" is distinguished from both chronic schizophrenia and dementia. The German psychiatrist Kraepelin, in 1919, used the term *paraphrenia* to classify a small group of his patients who exhibited marked paranoid delusions, yet maintained function in the community for months or even years. Paraphrenics were predominantly women and often lived alone. Even today, many of us can remember from childhood a single older woman who lived by herself in our neighborhood and rarely associated with other neighbors. She may have been considered strange in some of her behaviors, yet she continued to keep house, pay her bills, and maintain remarkably good health. A time often came, however, when she became increasingly suspicious, would not be heard from for days, and finally was forced to be taken to a hospital or a nursing home. Possibly she made frequent phone calls to the police reporting attacks by neighbors or strangers, none of which could be corroborated. The following description of such a woman is a current example of what Kraepelin described as late life paraphrenia.

 Mrs. Evans was 72 years old, single, and lived in a large house in a small North Carolina community. She was brought to psychiatric consultation by her niece (one of two living relatives) because of problems sleeping and an expressed fear that her in-laws were angry with her and were attempting retaliation for the settlement of her husband's estate. Mrs. Evans occasionally took in boarders to assist her financially, but had developed conflicts with these boarders (on almost every occasion) after two or three months.

Following the death of her husband twenty years prior to consultation, considerable conflict had arisen around the settlement of his estate. The family could not resolve the problem. Mrs. Evans and her sister-in-law each acquired a lawyer and a settlement was arranged. Though she rarely contacted her husband's family following the settlement, there had been no further challenges or problems from in-laws according to the patient's niece.

Mrs. Evans reported that she was experiencing a few physical problems, primarily arthritic. Her sleep had become sporadic, yet she attributed her sleep problems to visits by the in-laws at night, banging on the doors of her house and disturbing her. Although she sought help from her family and the police to prevent their intrusions, no one seemed to believe that the in-laws were "trying to drive me crazy." She protested that she had not been selfish in the settlement, yet her sister-in-law accused that she had not loved her husband but had lived with him only for his money. Her niece confirmed that such statements probably were made by the sister-in-law at the time of the settlement, but no angry words had been exchanged for years. As she described the legal settlement and the conflict to the psychiatrist, he had difficulty sorting through her reasoning as to why the in-laws had rekindled the old conflict. When pressed in the interview, Mrs. Evans admitted that she had not actually seen the in-laws during the night but had no question that they were banging on her door and shouting accusations at her. Though many college students living in the small town walked across her lawn and

neighborhood children played in her back yard, she was not troubled by
their presence nor had she suspected them to have participated in the
plot against her by her in-laws.

The psychiatrist found Mrs. Evans to be alert, oriented, and with no
evidence of problems with her memory or attention. Except for the
delusions (false beliefs) about her in-laws and hallucinations (hearing
voices), she did not appear particularly disturbed. The progress of her
thinking was logical (though unrealistic), she was friendly and in no
way felt threatened by the examination. A physical examination was
entirely normal except for an elevated blood pressure.

Mrs. Evans, a suspicious and withdrawn woman, exemplifies
late-life paraphrenia. In the United States, using our current diagnostic categories (see below), she would be diagnosed as suffering a
delusional disorder. No symptoms of schizophrenia were evident
except for the delusions regarding her in-laws and hallucinations
during the night. She continued to function at home, she was well
nourished, and she had no difficulty in relating to her neighbors. The
mental status examination failed to uncover any sign of a dementia.
She was treated with a low dose of an antipsychotic drug, thioridazine (Mellaril) and improved remarkably.

Suspiciousness and agitation may derive from a different
disorder in a very different context. The following case illustrates one
of the more common yet difficult problems faced by professionals
working with older adults.

Mrs. Arnold was first seen by a psychiatrist at the age of 64. She
complained of pain, nerves, and difficulty sleeping. For many years her
primary care physician had prescribed psychotherapeutic medications to
calm her "nerves." Because she focused on pain and sleep problems, she
refused to cooperate with psychological testing. The psychiatrist suspected
that she was suffering early memory loss, yet she was oriented to who
she was and where she was. As she had not responded to antidepressant
therapy and the sleep problems and agitation worsened, she was
prescribed electroconvulsive therapy (ECT). She did improve during these
treatments, but became confused with significant memory loss.

Two months after she had received the ECT treatments, she was less
confused but once again complained of pain and sleep problems.
Antidepressants were prescribed, but they were not effective. At the
encouragement of her daughter, she sought help from a number of

different psychiatrists during the following two years, all to no avail. Though she had occasional good days, she became an increasing burden upon her husband. She even began to accuse him of having an affair with another woman. Her accusations of infidelity were so disturbing to him that he sought psychiatric care for her as well as himself. At this time, she reluctantly agreed to psychological testing. Results revealed that she suffered significant focal impairments in memory and cognition. An MRI scan revealed multi-infarct dementia.

Despite the diagnosis, her husband wished to care for her at home, noting that he had promised never to have her institutionalized. She continued to see a local psychiatrist and was treated with an antipsychotic drug chlorpromazine (Thorazine). She slept reasonably well on the Thorazine, but during the day would become very agitated and physically attack her husband because of his infidelity. On two occasions she left the house and wandered through the neighborhood, found by the neighbors on one occasion and police on the other.

With time, she focused less upon her physical problems and more upon the maltreatment, infidelity, and stupidity of her husband. She even accused him of trying to poison her and beating her. He remained adamant that he would never institutionalize her, though he suffered bruises and became fearful that she might seriously injure him. Everyone who knew her was amazed at her strength and good physical health, despite the loss of memory and the psychotic behavior. Two months prior to her death she was institutionalized at the insistence of the family, for fear of the husband's safety. An autopsy confirmed the diagnosis of a multi-infarct dementia.

Some patients suffering a dementia are easily managed at home, whereas others suffer many psychiatric symptoms during the course of dementia, even to the point that the psychiatric symptoms dominate the clinical picture and cover the memory loss. In such cases, a complete diagnostic evaluation is difficult to accomplish given the uncooperativeness of the patient. A poor response to medications and ECT is, to some extent, diagnostic of a chronic dementing disorder leading to suspiciousness and agitation.

Disorders That Cause Suspiciousness and Agitation

Suspicious and agitated older adults, especially when the symptoms become severe, usually suffer from one of the following disorders. The first is a *chronic schizophrenic disorder* that persists from earlier in life into late life. As schizophrenia is characterized by a decline in function and a shorter life expectancy, chronic schizophrenia with persistent delusions is less likely to be found among the elderly than in mid-life. Some who suffer schizophrenia with severe symptoms in mid-life enter a quiescent period with improvement in their function and even remission from the illness. In others, the illness may reappear in the form of a delusional disorder. A decline in self-care activities usually distinguishes chronic schizophrenia from late life paraphrenia.

Another disorder is a late-onset schizophreniclike illness, often called *late life paraphrenia*, described above and illustrated in the case of Mrs. Evans (see page 90). Neither depression nor organic disorders contribute to these late-onset paranoid symptoms. Rather, late-onset schizophrenia is an autonomous disorder, chronic in its course, yet not leading to severe deterioration.

A disorder leading to suspiciousness and agitation is a *delusional disorder*. This disorder is not easily separated from late-onset schizophrenia, for the older person suffering a delusional disorder experiences delusions that he or she is being persecuted, especially by family and friends. These delusions usually center upon a single theme or possibly a series of connected themes. For example, an older man becomes convinced that a son is happy at the death of his mother (the older man's wife). The older man may have difficulty ever forgiving the child and much to the distress of the child, withdraw his affection, financial support, and limit social contact. Depressive symptoms are rare in such circumstances, yet agitation may accompany the disorder, often presenting as difficulty sleeping at night. The delusion is less bizarre than with late-onset schizophrenia and not accompanied by hallucinations.

Another disorder leading to delusions and suspiciousness is an *organic delusional syndrome*. The delusions, in contrast to a delusional disorder, are variable and wax and wane in severity. Delusions of persecution are the most common. These organic delusions may result from a number of factors, especially drug abuse (which is less common in older adults). The disease also may be secondary to damage to the temporal lobe of the brain or Huntington's chorea. For the patient to be diagnosed as suffering from an organic delusional syndrome, evidence must be found of brain disease that is responsible for the delusion. Organic hallucinations may accompany the delusions. Alcohol is the most common cause of an organic hallucination (and this syndrome is seen in late life as often as at other stages of the life cycle).

Finally, the *dementias* contribute to suspiciousness and agitation in late life. Both multi-infarct dementia and primary degenerative dementias of the Alzheimer's type precipitate restlessness and paranoid thoughts that dominate the clinical presentation, although a thorough evaluation reveals loss of memory. In contrast to the organic delusional disorder, these individuals rarely experience a loss of attention or clouding of consciousness. Loss of intellectual abilities (except for memory) is not prominent until late in the course and no other brain disease can be identified.

The Etiology of Suspiciousness and Agitation

Most investigators suspect cellular abnormalities as the predominant cause of suspiciousness and delusional thinking. Nevertheless, no specific biologic cause has been identified thus far. In rare cases, such as Huntington's chorea, a single genetic abnormality leads to brain disease that manifests symptoms similar to those of paranoid delusions in late life. A genetic abnormality is most likely not the cause of most late-life suspiciousness. A family history of suspiciousness and delusional thought is uncommon among persons suffering suspiciousness and agitation for the first time in late life.

The most accepted theory as to the cause of suspiciousness and agitation throughout the life cycle is the "dopamine theory." The nerve transmission system, which uses the chemical messenger dopamine, is hypothesized to be hyperactive in schizophrenia and delusional disorder. Evidence for hyperactivity of the dopamine system is largely circumstantial, however. A number of drugs are effective in reducing suspiciousness and delusional thinking, such as the antipsychotic drugs. The clinical effectiveness of these drugs is associated with their ability to attach to dopamine receptors in the brain. Levodopa (a drug used in the treatment of Parkinson's disease and which increases dopamine hyperactivity) will at times exacerbate the symptoms of schizophrenia, further supporting the dopamine hypothesis of schizophrenia.

A defect in brain function throughout the life cycle is thought to lead to abnormalities in the regulation of information transfer throughout the brain. Late-life schizophrenics are found to suffer degeneration at the base of the brain's cortex (the amygdala and hippocampus) and in the base of ganglia. Certain integrative psychophysiologic activities, such as the ability to follow moving objects with the eyes (eye tracking), are disrupted in schizophrenia. The resulting deficiency in maintaining attention and filtering information from the environment may lead to a hypervigilance and psychotic thinking.

These hypothesized abnormalities in attention lead to abnormal organization of thoughts, such as the "loss of ego boundaries." The paranoid and suspicious older adult loses a sense of where his or her own body and mind ends and where other minds and inanimate objects begin. For example, an older man may listen to the television and believe that an announcer is speaking directly to him. He may actually believe the announcer has entered into his head and is exerting an external influence.

These psychological abnormalities lead to three problems in thinking that are easily recognized. *Hallucinations* are false perceptions. Among suspicious older adults, these hallucinations are usually auditory (such as hearing a voice). *Illusions* (misinterpreted perceptions) may also be experienced by the suspicious and agitated older adult, especially if an organic delusional syndrome or a dementia is the cause of the suspiciousness. *Delusions* (false beliefs) are means by which the older adult organizes (albeit ineffectively) information that has been difficult to process. Although delusions may be bizarre and implausible, they organize stimuli in such a way that the older adult can explain the environment. When these false beliefs are challenged, agitation becomes a problem.

The family and social environment can also contribute to delusions. Isolated elders who seek to understand their surroundings often become confused. Not infrequently, older persons become disturbed that they are "cheating the government" because they have difficulty interpreting notices and forms sent by government agencies, such as those monitoring Medicare. A "warning letter" or some suggestion that a mistake has been made is interpreted as persecution from the outside and therefore precipitates paranoid thoughts.

The Diagnostic Workup

There are no available laboratory tests to diagnose the usual causes of suspiciousness and paranoid ideation in older adults. Even so, the laboratory workup is important to identify dysfunction at the organ and organ system levels in order to rule out the organic delusional syndrome. A chemistry screen, chest x ray, thyroid evaluation, and a blood count assist the clinician in identifying organic causes of the suspicious and paranoid behavior. Brain scan techniques such as computed axial tomography (CAT) or magnetic resonance imaging (MRI) may be of value in confirming the diagnosis of a dementia (especially a multi-infarct dementia) or in confirming evidence of shrinkage of parts of the brain in chronic schizophrenia. These imaging tests are not definitive and are therefore not required to properly care for uncomplicated suspiciousness. As suspiciousness is often associated with sensory impairment (especially difficulty seeing and hearing), audiometry and test of vision may identify potential areas for intervention.

The key to the diagnostic workup is the psychological evaluation. The nature of delusions and agitation is such that the patient's history more than likely will be inaccurate, thus making it important to interview the family to review the patient's behavior. Previous psychotic or delusional periods of behavior should be documented, as well as previous treatment (especially medications) administered to the patient for an emotional problem.

During the psychological evaluation, the clinician probes to determine whether the suspicious behavior is warranted. Older adults are occasionally abused. The convincing story of family members compared with a disorganized rambling of an elder suffering dementia makes this determination difficult. Nevertheless, clinicians must confront family members with accusations made by the older adult of either passive or active abuse. If following such a confrontation, the clinician is not convinced that the accusations are totally explained by the delusion, the social services department should be contacted.

In contrast, the older adult should not be challenged regarding the delusional thoughts. Opportunity should be provided for the elder to express his or her beliefs and feelings in an atmosphere of acceptance (though not necessarily agreement). The suspicious elder rarely insists that the clinicians (or others for that matter) agree with him. If asked to agree, the clinician should reply, "I don't understand the situation. When I complete my examination, I will try to make the best judgment I can. Regardless, I want to help you feel better and more secure. We both agree that you are upset, and that is the place to start." Such reassurance and attempts to ally in areas of agreement circumvent needless challenges to suspiciousness.

The evaluation of the family and social context of the delusional thinking is informed by the physical examination as much as by history. Evidence of physical abuse, neglect or trauma may appear in the form of bruises, poor hygiene of the skin, dehydration, or poor physical hygiene. An unkempt appearance does not necessarily reflect neglect by family members or caregivers. Rather, the suspicious and agitated older adult may have violently refused to bathe, dress properly, or eat meals prepared for him (because he may suspect the food to be poisoned). Concern for the health of the suspicious older adult often precipitates the referral for suspicious behavior to a clinician.

The clinician should also inquire as to the degree of agitation and disruption resulting from the suspicious and paranoid thinking. Has the older person physically attacked a family member or caregiver? Has the frightened or agitated state led to falls or other injuries? Does the older adult cooperate with medical management necessary for diseases such as diabetes and high blood pressure? Is the paranoid and suspicious elder disturbing others through behavior such as shouts or yells, temper tantrums, swearing, or cursing? Does the older person threaten others or endanger them by starting fights, arguments, threats, pushing people, or biting? Are there events or situations that precipitate suspicious or agitated behavior (such as the presence of someone who threatens the suspicious elder or changes such as a move)?

Treatment for Suspiciousness and Agitation

ENSURING A SAFE ENVIRONMENT

Prior to the initiation of the biopsychosocial treatment plan for the suspicious, agitated older adult, a decision must be made as to whether the elder should be managed as an outpatient or be hospitalized. Hospitalization may be necessary, but it should be considered only if outpatient therapy does not assure the security of the older person and the family. Paranoid elders do not adapt well to the hospital. A change in surroundings, interaction with persons who are unfamiliar, and the poorly understood activities of the hospital milieu each contribute to increases in suspiciousness and agitation. Suspicious elders will be reluctant to be admitted voluntarily and therefore require civil commitment to the hospital. Many hospitals, with legal clearance, have patients sign a 72-hour "voluntary commitment." If the older person changes his or her mind and wishes to be discharged before the treatment team determines that discharge is safe, then time is available to obtain an involuntary commitment. Such legal action against the paranoid elder appears, at first glance, extreme. Nevertheless, civil commitment is rarely disturbing or disruptive to the elder following recovery from acute and severe suspiciousness and agitation and should not be neglected if the safety and benefit of the elder are facilitated by commitment.

INITIATING A THERAPEUTIC ALLIANCE

Once the decision regarding location of treatment is made, the clinician must form an alliance with the suspicious elder. Suspicious older persons are (unlike younger schizophrenic patients) often lonely and seek companionship. Clinicians and other professionals are usually not included in the delusional thinking. The clinician, therefore, can take advantage of an initial acceptance by the patient to seek areas where a firm alliance can be formed. This therapeutic alliance is strengthened by identifying areas where the clinician and the patient can agree. If the older person agrees that he or she suffers a physical problem or anxiety (regardless of an interpretation of the cause of the anxiety) then empathy by the clinician for this problem fosters a willingness by the older adult to cooperate with therapy. As noted above, it is rarely necessary for the clinician to confront the elder regarding suspicious or delusional thinking. Responses to questions can be supportive, yet do not necessitate that the clinician agree with the paranoid elder.

PHARMACOLOGIC THERAPY

As the alliance is established, the clinician can begin treatment of the biologic abnormality. For nearly forty years, clinicians have used a powerful group of medications to treat suspiciousness and agitation—the antipsychotic or neuroleptic drugs. Chlorpromazine (Thorazine) was the first of these drugs available and is the primary reason the state hospital census is much lower today than it was fifty years ago. These drugs act by blocking a hypothesized hyperactive dopamine system, as described on page 94. In addition to chlorpromazine, other agents frequently used to treat older persons are thioridazine (Mellaril), haloperidol (Haldol), thiothixene (Navane) and more recently clozapine (Clozaril).

Antipsychotic drugs should be prescribed only when the symptoms of agitation and suspiciousness are severe enough that physical, psychological, and social functioning have deteriorated to the point that the results are distressing to the elder and/or dangerous to the elder or others. Even if the elder describes a bizarre delusion, when sleep is not disturbed and the elder continues to interact appropriately with the social environment, and self-care is not compromised, medications should not be prescribed. Antipsychotic drugs decrease the pressure of delusional and suspicious thinking and control agitation associated with such thoughts, but rarely lead to a "change of mind" regarding the delusion.

The physician selects the drug from this group based not only on the symptoms suffered but also side effects that are to be avoided (which differ from drug to drug). The dose of the drugs is generally lower than at earlier stages of life. The two most common drugs used in late life are also two of the most different, haloperidol and thioridazine. When the older person has difficulty sleeping, a low dose of thioridazine (10 to 25 mg at night) may be sufficient to improve sleep and to control suspiciousness and agitation. Thioridazine, however, can cause a drop in blood pressure upon standing (postural hypotension) and anticholinergic side effects such as a dry mouth.

IDENTIFYING THE IMMEDIATE CAUSES
OF AGITATION AND VIOLENT BEHAVIOR

The management of agitation and violent behavior does not consist of drug therapy alone. For a perspective on methods by which agitated and suspicious behavior can be controlled, professionals can best turn to the nursing literature, because the nursing profession is most often faced with the task of acute management of the aggressive patient.

Winger et al. (1987) catalog aggressive behavior into three categories. The first is disturbing behaviors, consisting of shouts or yells, angry outbursts, sarcastic remarks, swearing or cursing, and clenching or pounding one's fists. The second category is behaviors that endanger self, such as refusal of treatment, refusal to eat, refusal to follow directions, refusal to take medications, or overt opposition, such as doing the opposite of what is asked. The third category is behaviors that endanger others, such as hitting, pushing, beginning fights or arguments, threats of committing a violent act, breaking objects, pinching, and biting. In their study of approximately 170 patients with agitated behavior in a long-term care facility, Winger et al. found that 91 percent exhibited aggressive behavior. In most cases, there was a combination of the three categories, with 35 percent in the nursing home endangering self and disturbing others, and 40 percent endangering others, endangering self, and disturbing others. In an intermediate care facility, the percentage of individuals exhibiting aggressive behaviors decreased from 91 to 66 percent.

Boettcher (1983) suggested reasons for aggressive behavior:

- A need for territoriality (a comfortable space with freedom from crowding)
- A need for communication (to talk to a relative or a doctor)
- A need for self-esteem and freedom from insults or shame from others
- A need for safety/security (the elder strikes out in order to protect himself or herself)
- A need for authority (a need to have control)
- A need for one's own time (to move at one's own pace and not feel hurried)
- A need for personal identity (such as retention of personal items and identifying material)
- A need for comfort (to be free from physical or emotional pain)
- A need for cognitive understanding (an awareness of surroundings and orientation)

When these needs are not met, the elder experiences severe anxiety, which precipitates feelings of helplessness and entrapment and compels the elder to resort to behaviors which lead to some mastery or control over these feelings, regardless of their maladaptive outcome.

CONTROLLING VIOLENT BEHAVIOR

Morton (1987) suggests the following guidelines for minimizing the risk and controlling violent behavior. Appreciate that the physical aggression represents an attempt to achieve security and control. Any intervention, therefore, should, if possible, lead to an increased sense of security by the elder rather than a sense of entrapment and external control. For example, if the patient can be provided with more responsibility, then violence may be decreased.

Avoid taking the patient's verbal and physical abuse personally. Nursing staff and aides, as well as physicians, should recognize that the verbal abuse received from patients within a long-term care facility is not directed at them. Nevertheless, a continual barrage of abusive language can lead to retaliation. Nurses are the usual convenient targets of pent-up emotions of the distraught elder. It is important to remain objective, recognize the cursing and abuse for what it is, and, at all costs, avoid any retaliative behaviors. A similar approach applies outside medical facilities.

Physical struggle is time-limited. Even though the strength of a suspicious and aggressive elder may appear to be incredibly persistent, intense physical struggle cannot be sustained indefinitely. Therefore, the immediate task is to minimize risk and injury to both patient and staff during the time of an assault. Recognize the importance of teamwork. Strength alone is not the only factor that can maintain an advantage in a physical struggle with a suspicious older adult. Most suspicious elders act impulsively and erratically, relying on physical force alone. The medical and nursing staff, in contrast, can plan their approach and overcome the physical strength of the elder with a logical and sequential approach to intervention.

Recognize that effective management of aggressive behavior begins by taking three critical steps:

1. Accurately evaluate the situation and the best intervention.
2. Get help as soon as possible and avoid a physical struggle between a patient and a single member of the medical or nursing staff (one-on-one struggles increase the risk of injury to both parties).
3. Develop a plan utilizing the staff that assembles them in the crisis situation.

Appreciate that rising levels of emotions in both the patient and staff result during a physical assault, regardless of staff training and preparation. As quickly as possible, implement techniques to diminish the intensity of the emotions of both staff and patients.

PREVENTING VIOLENT BEHAVIOR

According to Morton (1986), when suspicion leads to increased emotional tension and threats of aggression, the nursing staff can intervene to decrease tension in the following ways.

1. Psychologically disarm the threatening patient by expressing his or her anxiety verbally. Say things such as, "Mrs. Smith, you appear to be very upset. I am Mr. Jones, your attendant, and I want to help you." Encourage the patient to express his or her anger verbally. When the interactions are kept at a verbal level and taken seriously, tension usually decreases within a short time.

2. Direct the attention of the disturbed elder. In times of stress, the elder (possibly confused secondary to a physical illness) cannot distinguish the variety of stimuli encroaching upon her from the environment. One staff member should calmly speak to the elder and serve as a single source of communication. By continually repeating the name of the disturbed elder, behavior can be better controlled.

3. Give directions for even the most simple of behaviors. The suspicious and disturbed elder has difficulty in making complex decisions and adaptive responses. Therefore, the clinician should say, "Mr. Smith, turn loose of my arm. Now sit in the chair. We are going to talk."

4. Communicate clearly and concisely. Short simple statements enable the elder suffering a decreased ability to receive and organize information to process verbal stimuli and respond more appropriately.

5. Communicate expectations. Staff should be clear when they approach the patient and request the elder to do something. For example, "Mrs. Smith, sit down and do not throw any more objects. You cannot leave the room. If you want something, ask for it, and I will bring it to you."

6. Avoid arguing or defending. When the suspicious elder suspects that he or she has frightened or angered a staff member, this heightens anxiety and increases defensive behavior on the part of the elder.

7. Avoid threatening body language. In intense situations, it is tempting for staff to clinch their fists, cross their hands over their chests, and to make quick and rapid movements. Instead, staff should move slowly and model a behavior that can be adapted by the disturbed and suspicious elder.

8. Respect personal space. The suspicious and aggressive elder should not be approached closely. If possible, staff should keep as much distance as feasible until the elder has been calmed.

FURTHER DEVELOPING
THE THERAPEUTIC ALLIANCE

Once agitated and aggressive behaviors are controlled, professionals can once again attempt to develop a therapeutic relationship with the suspicious elder (Blazer and Hamrick, 1984). Unlike younger people, the elderly patient who is psychotic yet not agitated will usually accept physicians and other professionals as friends and even confidants. They will openly express their own fears, concerns, and beliefs about what is happening to them with no fear that the professional will discredit their statements or disagree. Therefore, it is important for the professional to take an interest in the patient; for instance, a physician can take a medical interest. Areas of agreement should be sought in conversation to support the therapeutic alliance.

The professional, however, should not agree with the unwarranted suspicions of the elder in order to establish a relationship. A dishonest approach to a suspicious elder will lead to conflict. The professional should also avoid attacking or attempting to change the mind of the suspicious elder. Rational arguments are rarely beneficial. Although the suspicious elder rarely asks a professional, "Do you believe what I am telling you?" he or she does want some assurance that the professional will not discredit or abuse him or her.

The following approach is of value in developing a therapeutic relationship with the suspicious elder (Blazer and Hamrick, 1984):

- Take a medical orientation (an area where both professional and elder can agree).
- Interview the suspicious elder on his or her territory (at home if possible).
- Remain courteous, attentive, open, and interested.
- Be honest, neutral, and consistent.
- Do not agree with the suspicious elder about hallucinatory thoughts or delusions.
- Empathize with the patient in his or her feelings.
- Encourage the suspicious elder to discuss mistrust openly.
- Assist the suspicious elder in avoiding large groups (which usually heighten suspiciousness).

WORKING WITH THE FAMILY OF THE SUSPICIOUS AND AGITATED ELDER

Family members often receive the brunt of paranoid thoughts emanating from a suspicious older adult and, not infrequently, also are the victims of their violent outbursts. Therefore, families can greatly benefit from the assistance of professionals as follows (Blazer and Hamrick, 1984):

- Identify the family members or friends whom the patient trusts.
- Always talk with the suspicious elder first when the elder is brought to the office by family members.
- Interview family members alone only with the elder's permission.
- Do not side with the family in the suspicious elder's presence.
- Limit the number of sessions with family members alone to those sessions that are absolutely necessary so that the suspicious elder does not suspect collusion between the professional and the family.
- Encourage the family to express their frustration, fears, and guilt.
- Alleviate family frustrations by emphasizing the difficulty in managing the suspicious elder.

- Educate the family into techniques for managing abusive language and even physical outbursts.
- Alleviate family fears by explaining the origin and expected outcome of the suspicious elder's condition.
- Suggest practical means by which the family can interact with the suspicious elder (these same techniques used by the professional and described above).

References

Blazer, D. G., and A. Hamrick, "Paranoid disorders." In D. G. Blazer and I. C. Siegler (Eds.), *A Family Approach to Health Care in the Elderly.* Menlo Park, CA: Addison-Wesley Publishing Co., 1984. Pp. 205–221.

Boettcher, E. G. "Preventing violent behavior." *Perspectives in Psychiatric Care*, 21:54, 1983.

Christenson, R., and D. G. Blazer. "Epidemiology of persecutory ideation in an elderly population in the community." *American Journal of Psychiatry*, 141:1088, 1984.

Lowenthal, M. F. *Lives in Distress.* New York: Basic Books, 1964.

Morton, P. "Managing." *American Journal of Nursing*, 25:1114–1116, 1986.

Winger, J. Schirmv, and D. Stewart. "Aggressive behavior in long-term care." *Journal of Psychosocial Nursing*, 25:28, 1987.

Suggested Reading

Christison, C. G., and D. G. Blazer. "Late-life schizophrenia and paranoid disorders." In E. W. Busse and D. G. Blazer (Eds.), *Geriatric Psychiatry.* Washington, DC: American Psychiatric Press, 1989. Pp. 403–414.

Jeste, D. V., and S. Zisook (Eds.). "Psychosis and depression in the elderly." *The Psychiatric Clinics of North America*, 11:1, 1988.

Miller, N. E., and J. D. Cohen (Eds.). *Schizophrenia and Aging: Schizophrenia, Paranoia, and Schizophreniform Disorders in Later Life.* New York: The Gilford Press, 1987.

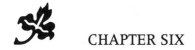

CHAPTER SIX

Anxiety

Anxiety is among the more common problems experienced across the life cycle. Though the "age of anxiety" described by W. H. Auden (1946) during the years of World War II has been replaced, according to some, by the "age of melancholy," anxiety continues to be a major malady of our time. Worry may arise about one's health, personal loss, the future, economic security, or spontaneously with no clear explanation as to why the elder is worried. Regardless of origin, severe and persistent anxiety, not infrequently associated with episodes of panic, can be disabling to an otherwise healthy older adult. Many related emotional problems are accompanied by worry, such as phobic disorders, obsessive-compulsive disorders, and anxiety secondary to physical illness.

Survey researchers in Kentucky discovered that 17 percent of males and 21 percent of females in a representative community sample of persons over the age of 55 reported sufficient anxiety symptoms to be judged candidates for some form of therapy (Himmelfarb and Murrell, 1984). Persons in urban counties, low in social and economic status, and with a lower education were found to have the highest prevalence of anxiety. In a similar study, but with more restrictive criteria for clinically significant anxiety, the one-year prevalence of generalized anxiety among persons 65 years of age and older was nearly 3 percent, similar to the prevalence at other stages of the life cycle. In both of these studies, anxiety was related to poor physical health (Blazer et al., in press).

The presentation of the emotional problems of anxiety and worry is illustrated by the following cases of older persons.

Mrs. Jensen was a 77-year-old woman who came to visit her primary care physician at the insistence of her daughter. For twenty years she had suffered from "nerves," dating approximately to the time that she retired from her work as a cashier in a supermarket. Though always the nervous type, worry and anxiety had increased gradually since her retirement. She had seen a physician five years before who had prescribed the nerve medicine diazepam (Valium) and she had taken the medicine intermittently when she felt especially anxious.

During the months prior to seeing the doctor, she had suffered more symptoms of dizziness. When the dizzy spells occurred, her heart would race and she would feel prickling around her lips, pain in her chest, and shortness of breath. Though the dizzy episodes only lasted for a few seconds, she began to worry that her heart was failing. She felt as if her heart was about to jump out of her chest. On one occasion, she even imagined that she had suffered a small stroke. When examined in the physician's office, he found no evidence of disease in her heart or in her blood pressure. Her neurologic examination was normal. He suggested she continue to take the Valium when needed. She returned a few months later, saying that she had continued to take Valium in about the same amount as she had in the past but she could feel no evidence that the medicine was of benefit. She finally chose to stop taking Valium, and had discontinued the drug for a month before the return visit. She suffered no increase in her symptoms and the dizziness was not as much of a problem as previously.

Mrs. Jensen experienced symptoms of a mild panic disorder. The panic attacks were frequent, occurring every two to three days, but they were not associated with specific fears. She carried out her usual activities despite the attacks. Though always "nervous," she had learned to live with the episodes of panic. The treatment of panic disorders with medications (as described below) is only of moderate benefit. When elders such as Mrs. Jensen do not recognize a benefit from the drug, it is usually best that they discontinue taking the drug. Periodic evaluation by her physician was sufficient to monitor the symptoms of panic.

Mr. Barnes had suffered anxiety in the mornings for approximately one year. He suspected his problems began when he decided to place his mother in a nursing home (she was 93) and sell the "home place," which had been in the family for over 100 years. His mother, who had become incapable of caring for herself, would need the money from the sale to provide her with adequate nursing care for the remaining years of her life.

Mr. Barnes' mother was suffering some memory difficulties and had always depended upon her son, especially during her later years. She was agreeable to the move and enjoyed her friends there. Nevertheless, Mr. Barnes remembered a promise he made to his mother many years before—that he would never place her in a "home." Her daily care, however, required more than he and his wife were capable of providing. He visited his mother each day in the nursing home and she welcomed his visits. Six months after admission to the home, however, she suffered a severe stroke and, after being hospitalized, returned to the nursing home. She was unable to communicate upon her return. Mr. Barnes could not even be certain that his mother knew him following the stroke.

The anxiety experienced by Mr. Barnes occurred predominantly in the early mornings when he would awake, lie in bed, and reminisce regarding his past life (especially about his mother). He recognized a pattern to his symptoms. If he would get out of bed soon after awakening, the anxiety could be alleviated. Once he was out of bed and moving around (especially after he had taken his early morning walk), the anxiety disappeared. Through the remainder of the day, he rarely suffered from anxiety.

Mr. Barnes improved after four sessions with a local psychologist, who helped him recognize the source of his anxiety—a fear that he was not being a supportive and loving son to his mother. When Mr. Barnes appraised the situation, he recognized the many years of effort directed toward maintaining his mother at home. He also recognized that the humane care she was receiving in the nursing home could not be provided at home. Four months after Mr. Barnes was initially evaluated, his mother died. He grieved her death during the following two months and began to focus upon the excellent relationship he had with his mother over the years. The anxiety decreased and he found himself more engaged in his retirement interests.

Mr. Barnes suffered from an adjustment disorder with anxious mood. The anxiety that he suffered in the mornings was a reaction to placing his mother in a nursing home. The symptoms were relatively brief in duration and when his mother died, he was convinced that he had done everything possible to alleviate her suffering.

Disorders That Cause Anxiety

The anxiety disorders encompass emotional problems that either result from attempts to control anxiety (such as the phobic disorders) or responses that exaggerate anxiety (such as panic disorder). The distinguishing characteristic of a *generalized anxiety disorder* is an unrealistic or excessive worry and anxiety about problems in one's life, such as worry about grandchildren, finances, physical health, or living conditions (APA, 1987). When the symptoms of anxiety are associated with worry only in one area and the worry is realistic, the older adult should not be labeled as suffering from generalized anxiety. Symptoms of generalized anxiety can be categorized as follows: autonomic hyperactivity, such as shortness of breath, sweating, palpitations, and dizziness; motor tension, such as trembling and restlessness; and hypervigilance, such as feeling keyed up or on edge, having difficulty falling asleep or being excessively frightened when surprised. Anxiety symptoms are often a component of many emotional problems afflicting older adults (such as the agitation and anxiety accompanying major or clinical depressions) and therefore the diagnosis of generalized anxiety should only be applied when other causes of the anxiety have been eliminated.

Panic disorder has received much attention in recent years, although panic is much less common among older adults than generalized anxiety. Fewer than 1 percent of older adults suffer episodes of panic frequent enough to be classified as suffering from a panic disorder. The anxious symptoms that accompany a panic disorder usually derive from the fear of suffering another panic attack. Attacks of panic are characterized by shortness of breath (even a sense of smothering), dizziness, sweating, depersonalization or derealization (e.g., feelings of unreality, such as observing oneself from outside), tingling in the hands and feet, and chest pain. The onset of panic can occur at any time, though panic at night is rare (usually when the elder awakens from a frightening dream). No cause of the panic, such as a frightening experience, can usually be identified (APA, 1987).

Obsessive-compulsive disorder is characterized by recurrent obsessions or compulsions that are severe enough to cause distress and consuming enough to interfere with the normal social functioning (APA, 1987). When the elder cannot continue his or her compulsive activities, anxiety usually results. Obsessions are persistent thoughts or images that are intrusive, threatening, or senseless (such as thoughts by a devoted husband that he should be having an affair). Compulsions are purposeful and repetitive behaviors that are performed in a stereotypic fashion in order to neutralize the discomfort of anxiety. Unlike panic disorder, obsessive compulsive disorder is just as common in late life as in young adulthood.

Phobic disorders are among the most common disorders affecting persons in late life and may be accompanied by anxiety and panic. Researchers are not sure why this is so. One of the more severe phobias is agoraphobia, the fear of being in places or situations from which escape would be difficult or at least embarrassing (APA, 1987). For example, the older person may fear being in a crowd (such as sitting in a religious assembly) and therefore may avoid lifelong activities in order to avoid the fear of being trapped in the crowd. Older persons suffering from panic and agoraphobia usually restrict travel and often require a companion when away from home. Situations that are especially problematic for the agoraphobic are fears of being outside the home alone, traveling on a bus, a train, or an automobile or standing in line. When severe, the agoraphobic will not leave the house, or even a room in the house.

Another disorder that may lead to symptoms of anxiety is the *organic anxiety syndrome* (APA, 1987). Organic anxiety may be caused by problems with endocrine function such as excessive production of thyroid hormone, low blood sugar (hypoglycemia) or, in rare cases, a tumor (pheochromocytoma). Intoxication from stimulants ranging from caffeine to the amphetamines or withdrawal from substances that depress the central nervous system, such as sleeping pills and alcohol, also may cause an organic anxiety syndrome.

The Etiology of Anxiety

Fear and anxiety are analogous but distinct emotional states. When an older woman must walk home through a dangerous neighborhood after shopping, she experiences fear from the moment she departs the store until she reaches the safety of her apartment. The distress and discomfort is acute, yet appropriate to the situation. In contrast, the older woman who feels as anxious and uncomfortable in her home as when walking in the street experiences a slow and chronic distress that cannot be logically attributed to the situation. What is the origin of this fear that has no focus?

In recent years, biologic theories of anxiety have predominated as increased understanding of anxiety emerges in a rapidly developing area of clinical and basic investigation (Barlow, 1988). A number of chemical messengers (neurotransmitters) have been implicated as involved in the etiology of anxiety. GABA (gamma-aminobutyric acid) is the principal chemical messenger that inhibits transmission of information from one nerve cell to another in the central nervous system. The medications that are most frequently used for treating anxiety, the benzodiazepines, increase the activity of GABA by increasing the affinity of the chemical messenger for its binding site. Unfortunately, the chemical messenger GABA is difficult to study in humans and therefore little is known regarding differences in the concentration or action of the messenger across the life cycle.

Another chemical messenger frequently implicated in anxiety is norepinephrine (noradrenalin). Drugs that affect norepinephrine, such as the tricyclic antidepressants, are effective in treating the more severe anxiety disorders (panic attacks). Norepinephrine originates in a nucleus at the base of the brain called the locus ceruleus, which is thought to decrease in activity with increased age. Nevertheless, the decreased activity of the production of norepinephrine could be offset by increased sensitivity of the brain to norepinephrine with aging.

At the organ and organ system level, the symptoms of anxiety parallel a system dysfunction known as autonomic hyperactivity. In the hyperactive state, the autonomic nervous system (that part of the nervous system not under the control of the person) produces an increased heart rate, increased sweating, decreased blood flow to the stomach (often causing cramps), and flushing—

those very changes in the body that prepare the body to respond to a challenge (the fight or flight response). If hyperactivity persists, then the older adult suffers a chronic and excessive overload of stimulation and therefore suffers generalized anxiety or even panic.

The psychological theories of anxiety have been most extensively elaborated by the psychoanalytic school of Sigmund Freud. He theorized that anxiety is a signal to the consciousness that an unacceptable impulse or drive is pushing to become conscious. Anxiety in turn arouses the ego to take some measure to protect against the conscious representation of the drive or memory. For example, with Mr. Barnes, the unconscious desire to place his mother in a facility where he could be free to do what he wished and not be burdened with her care signaled anxiety, for he could not consciously retract his promise never to put her in a nursing home. That placing his mother in a long-term care facility was the rational decision did not alleviate the signal anxiety from the unconscious drives. Anxiety in such circumstances may be manifest in anxious symptoms or may be controlled by defensive behaviors such as compulsive acts or displacement of the anxiety upon an identified object (leading to phobia).

Other investigators have proposed that learning is central to the development of anxiety across the life cycle (Marks, 1978). Anxiety is a conditioned response to stimuli from the environment. The older person may become dizzy after taking a new blood pressure medication. The dizzy spell has no relation to the medication, yet the older person associates dizziness with taking medication. Through the process of generalization, the elder begins to distrust all medications, believing they will lead to dizziness. Anxiety increases when the physician and family members encourage the older person that the medication is necessary to control a chronic mental illness.

At the psychosocial and cultural level, anxiety may arise in older persons who reflect upon their lives and their positions in society (if not the universe). For no apparent reason, the older person becomes profoundly aware of a sense of "nothingness" or insignificance in life. Such overwhelming anxiety may be more disturbing than the fear of death. Existential anxiety may accompany and exaggerate anxiety from other sources and should not be ignored by professionals working with older adults. Rather, professionals should, when appropriate, collaborate with the clergy who minister to the elder or with a hospital or institutional chaplain, or encourage discussion with other elders with similar beliefs and values.

The Diagnostic Workup

One laboratory test that has been used on occasion to help identify the biologic contribution to panic is the lactate infusion test. Because individuals suffering anxiety do not tolerate overexertion, they produce more lactate than normal. Lactate is a product of the energy cycle that can produce muscle cramps. The test involves intravenously administering a solution of sodium lactate to an older adult who is in good physical health but appears to be suffering panic attacks. Over 70 percent of individuals suffering true panic disorder (but only 5 percent of normals) will develop a panic attack when they receive the lactate infusion. Panic under such a circumstance suggests the potential success of a biologic intervention such as medication.

Physical examination reveals evidence of autonomic hyperactivity and endocrine abnormalities associated with anxiety. If the elder's thyroid hormone production is elevated, his or her eyes may protrude (exophthalamos), the thyroid gland may be enlarged (producing a bulge at the front of the neck), and the hands may be tremulous. Reflexes are more brisk than normal. Careful examination of the heart in an individual suffering autonomic hyperactivity reveals a rapid heart rate and greater changes in heart rate on some activity (such as standing). Skin often is warm and moist and the face may be flushed.

The clearest evidence for an anxiety disorder with accompanying symptoms (such as obsessions, compulsions, and phobias) comes once again from the clinical interview. Most older persons spontaneously reveal the discomfort of subjective anxiety. A review with the elder and family members permits the clinician to distinguish generalized anxiety from anxiety associated with panic. Symptoms of obsessions and compulsions should be explored (such as ritualistic behavior, unwanted thoughts, and irrational acts). Those behaviors and thoughts that are abnormal to the clinician, however, may be accepted as perfectly normal by the older adult (such as checking the lock twice before leaving the house). The older person should be asked about fears (whether they are perceived as unrealistic or not) and to what extent these fears interfere with usual activities. If the person is suffering chronic anxiety and panic attacks, a careful review of prescription and nonprescription medications is imperative. Excessive caffeine intake or the use of other stimulants is important to identify. Many elders do not connect anxiety with the three or four cups of coffee they drink in the morning.

During the mental status examination, the clinician must first rule out the presence of cognitive impairment and an attentional disorder secondary to delirium. Delirium with agitation is difficult to distinguish from panic attack. Clinicians must be persistent, calm, and unhurried when examining the elder if the mental status examination is to be successful with the anxious older adult. Significant anxiety can interfere with the performance of tasks during cognitive testing, especially calculations (such as asking a person to perform simple mathematical tasks).

The setting of anxiety is important to establish in order to determine if actual psychosocial events are contributing to the symptoms of anxiety. Do the symptoms of anxiety change from place to place or at different times throughout the day? Many older persons become anxious in the mornings, when the house is quiet or when they are awakened because of a sound on the street. The symptoms of anxiety must also be set within the context of the life history and life view of the older adult. A crisis in the life of the older adult may have little to do with physical functioning or even immediate psychological or psychosocial difficulties. Rather, the older person may suffer an existential crisis regarding his or her religious beliefs, perception of contribution to society, or the state of affairs of a world that is soon to be departed.

Treatment for Anxiety

Anxiety is contagious. Professionals who attempt to treat elders suffering anxiety may experience a sense of panic and urgency themselves. The older adult experiencing anxiety emits a message to "do something" as quickly as possible. Inappropriate efforts to relieve the anxiety, however, precipitate more problems than they correct. Therefore, the first step in treating the anxious older adult is to take a calm and deliberate approach to the therapeutic challenge.

Despite the severe discomfort that anxiety produces, the anxious patient can tolerate these symptoms for minutes, hours, and even days. Permitting the older adult to ventilate the severity of the symptoms in a calm setting to an interested and receptive clinician often eliminates the sense of the emergency when treating the anxious older adult.

PHARMACOLOGIC THERAPY

If acute and severe anxiety afflicts an older adult, judicious use of antianxiety drugs is indicated. The benzodiazepines are the most frequently used medications for treating anxiety. Two drugs are used more often than any others and reflect the differences between the various benzodiazepines—diazepam (Valium) and alprazolam (Xanax). All of the benzodiazepine antianxiety agents, when used in appropriate dosage, can reduce the subjective sense of anxiety without producing unwanted sedation, confusion, and disorientation. Despite adverse publicity, these drugs usually do not cause severe side effects. For this reason, as much as any other, the drugs are used widely and prescribed frequently by primary care physicians, yet benzodiazepines can be addicting, especially when used in excessive doses over long periods of time. The most common problematic side effects from long-term and excessive use of the benzodiazepines are difficulty with balance, slowed reaction time, slurring of speech, and insomnia. These effects can be exaggerated by other medications (such as some antihypertensive drugs and alcohol).

Diazepam (Valium) is the most frequently used of the antianxiety agents, or at least it has been for the past twenty years, with a usual dose of 2 to 5 mg once or twice a day. The drug is relatively long acting. After ingestion, it reaches its maximum blood level within two to three hours and has a half-life of 12 to 24 hours. The length of action of a drug after being ingested is usually measured by the number of hours from ingestion until one-half of the drug is eliminated from the bloodstream. The elimination half-life of diazepam is three times longer in older persons compared to younger adults. Effects of the medication may persist in an older adult for days following the last dose. For this reason, an antianxiety drug with a shorter half-life is usually preferred in treating the elderly.

The most commonly used of these agents today is alprazolam (Xanax). The usual dose of alprazolam is between 0.25 and 1 mg two to three times per day. Peak blood levels are reached within 30 minutes after taking the drug and the significant effects usually have subsided two to three hours after the drug is taken. For this reason, older persons may experience a rebound of symptoms a few hours after taking a short-acting antianxiety agent and therefore may increase the daily dose of the drug by taking it more frequently. Older adults who take a short-acting antianxiety agent like alprazolam at night may not have difficulty falling asleep but may find themselves awakening two to three hours into the night suffering rebound anxiety. All of the benzodiazepine antianxiety drugs can lead to confusion and, if taken in high enough doses, problems with balance and coordination. They also can be addictive, although the risk for addiction is low.

Other medications are prescribed to persons for treating anxiety, most of which are of value in particular situations. Hydroxyzine (Vistaril, Atarax) is a safe drug similar to the antihistamines that may be prescribed during the day. Unlike the benzodiazepines, hydroxyzine does not lead to addiction or tolerance. The subjective decrease in anxiety, however, is less apparent than with the benzodiazepines. A new drug recently introduced to the market is buspirone (Buspar). As with hydroxyzine, buspirone does not lead to addiction or tolerance. Buspirone is well tolerated by older adults but probably is of use only for patients who suffer "chronic tension." For individuals who experience periodic episodes of panic or situational anxiety, buspirone is of little value.

For persons suffering anxiety in predictable situations (such as speaking before a group of people), the drug propranolol (Inderal) is useful for relieving the physical symptoms of anxiety, such as palpitations, urinary frequency, rapid heart rate, and tremor. Propranolol is usually used for treating high blood pressure. The drug has little effect on "psychic" anxiety. An older person forced into a stressful situation (such as speaking to a group of elders) can take 10 mg of propranolol thirty minutes before the stressful situation and can tolerate the anxiety precipitated by the situation. Use of the drug in this way must be judicious. In severe cases of anxiety and agitation, antipsychotic drugs such as haloperidol can be used to treat anxiety. These drugs are described more fully on pages 98–99.

The primary treatment of panic disorder is the use of anti-depressant agents, especially the tricyclic antidepressants. Imipramine is the drug that has been most frequently used to treat panic throughout the life cycle. It is given in a dose similar to that given for treating a clinical or major depression. Because the drug may not be tolerated as well in an anxious older adult, the increase in dosage to a maximum dose level should be slower than in treating someone younger who is suffering a severe depression. As with depression, 2½ to 5 weeks may be required to control the panic disorder.

When the tricyclic antidepressants are ineffective, the monoamine oxidase inhibitors (MAOIs) may be used. A new drug called clomipramine (a tricyclic antidepressant) has been found to be especially effective in treating obsessive compulsive disorder. The drug is not yet available in the United States (except in specialized research centers), but it should be marketed in the near future. This drug represents a significant pharmacologic breakthrough in treating the treatment-resistant obsessive compulsive disorders.

PSYCHOTHERAPY

The psychotherapy of the anxiety disorders is generally directed at reducing the sense of helplessness in the anxious elder and enhancing a sense of control. Such control can be effected by teaching the older adult to control body function. Biofeedback is one means by which anxiety can be controlled. Most biofeedback procedures are based on the theory that the autonomic nervous system is not autonomous but rather can be controlled by conscious attempts to relax. Some type of electronic amplification of physiologic symbols serves as feedback to the patient through sight or sound. For example, sweating of the skin can be fed back through a visual signal and the elder can, through relaxation techniques learned through biofeedback, lower the tendency to sweat. In other situations, muscle tension (for instance, in the neck or forehead) is fed back to the elder who responds by lowering the tension in these muscles.

Persons throughout the life cycle have exhibited an ability to control a number of so-called autonomous functions through biofeedback techniques, including rate of blood flow, bladder function, heart rate, and blood pressure. Although older persons are thought to be able to learn such responses less quickly than the young, an alert and motivated elder can be successful at traditional biofeedback techniques, regardless of age.

Biofeedback is usually paired with other therapies, especially training in relaxation. Relaxation training can be a benefit to older persons as it can to persons at other stages of life. The elder is instructed in relaxing different sets of muscles throughout the body, usually beginning with the extremities and working up the trunk to control of breathing, tension in the jaw, and so forth. The elder is instructed to substitute pleasant and relaxing thoughts for frightening or anxiety-provoking thoughts.

Psychotherapy is of less benefit for treating the anxiety disorders than pharmocologic therapy or behavior therapy (Gorman and Liebowitz, 1987). It should not be ignored, however, as a potential aid, especially in alleviating generalized anxiety. Psychotherapy has little therapeutic benefit for older persons suffering panic disorder or obsessive compulsive disorder, except that the educational approach to therapy enables the older adult to understand the nature of the problem and, therefore, the perceived severity of the disorder (such as the fear that one is having a heart attack) can be alleviated. Psychotherapists often search in vain to find symbolic meanings for anxiety and panic. Though associations may exist, identification of these associations in therapy has been of little benefit, except in less severe cases of anxiety. For example, in the case of Mr. Barnes, a better understanding of his mother's condition and his reaction to her condition was of benefit. Nevertheless, it was only after the death of his mother and the resolution of his grief around her death that the symptoms of anxiety actually abated.

Psychotherapy generally should be directed toward helping the older adult assume greater control over his or her environment. This control can be facilitated through the therapist-patient relationship. The therapist should encourage patients to participate actively in the therapeutic contract (such as determining the number of therapy sessions, the goals of therapy, and the topics to be discussed in the session). As anxiety is often associated with concerns about physical health and body integrity, the therapist can be of great assistance to the elder in providing information regarding the nature and extent of whatever physical problems are suffered. Even if such explanations are of no benefit in actually improving the elder's health, a greater understanding of the illness (such as the mechanisms by which diabetes can lead to visual problems) can decrease anxiety.

Clinicians can do much to decrease anxiety about the patient's environment. Encouragement to become involved in simple, repetitive tasks that do not require a deadline or appreciable problem solving (such as gardening or quilting) help dissipate energy and increase relaxation. Clinicians should work with elders to identify their interests, even making a list of their activities that are appropriate to the time of year and situation. Interests and attention span for given activities should be determined. Clinicians can assist the elder in developing a daily schedule that is not too rigorous or demanding, yet provides enough activity that the older person is at less risk for sitting a number of hours and fostering increased anxiety during this time.

Family members should be alert to the nature of the anxiety disorder suffered by the older adult and ways in which they may assist in decreasing the anxiety. Relatives should especially be alerted to the feelings of helplessness and lack of control experienced by many elders suffering generalized anxiety by anticipating the needs of such elders and intervening before the situation becomes a crisis, which precipitates severe anxiety. Such crisis intervention may especially be of value in alleviating the anxiety that derives from decreased orientation secondary to early memory loss.

References

American Psychological Association. *Diagnostic and Statistical Manual of Mental Disorders* (3d ed.). Washington, DC: American Psychological Association, 1987.

Auden, W. H. *The Age of Anxiety.* New York: Random House, 1946.

Barlow, D. H. *Anxiety and Its Disorders: The Nature and Treatment of Anxiety and Panic.* New York: Guilford Press, 1988.

Blazer, D. G., D. Hughes, L. K. George, M. Swartz, and J. Boyer. "Generalized anxiety disorders." In L. N. Robins and D. Reiger (Eds.), *Psychiatric Disorders in America.* New York: Free Press, in press.

Gorman, J. M., and M. R. Liebowitz. "Panic and anxiety disorders." In R. Michaels and J. O. Cavenar (Eds.), *Psychiatry*, Volume 1. Philadelphia: J. B. Lippincott, 1987.

Himmelfarb, S., and S. A. Murrell. "The prevalence and correlates of anxiety symptoms in older adults." *The Journal of Psychology*, 116:159-167, 1984.

Marks, I. M. "Behavioral psychotherapy of adult neurosis." In *The Handbook of Psychotherapy and Behavioral Change*. New York: John Wiley and Sons, 1978.

Suggested Reading

Bergman, N. N. K. "Neurosis and personality disorder in old age." In A. D. Isaacs and F. Post (Eds.), *Studies in Geriatric Psychiatry*. New York: John Wiley and Sons, 1978.

Brickman, A. L., and C. Eisdorfer. "Anxiety in the elderly." In E. W. Busse and D. G. Blazer (Eds.), *Geriatric Psychiatry*. Washington, DC: American Psychiatric Press, 1989. Pp. 415–428.

Pies, R. "Differential diagnosis of anxiety in the elderly." *Geriatric Medicine Today*, 5:94, 1986.

Saltzman, C. "Treatment of anxiety disorders." In C. Saltzman (Ed.), *Clinical Geriatric Psychopharmacology*. New York: McGraw-Hill, 1984. Pp. 132–148.

CHAPTER SEVEN

Hypochondriasis and Other Somatoform Disorders

Hypochondriasis in older adults is one of the more common and frustrating somatoform problems encountered by professionals. The problem, although exhibiting itself as biologic or medical, is actually psychological and invariably affects the interaction of the older adult with family members, friends, and especially health care providers. Physicians encounter patients who come to the office complaining of multiple problems without apparent illness and family members or friends sit for hours listening to a symptom recital from the hypochondriacal elder.

Although these patients could benefit from counseling from a psychiatrist or other mental health worker, they rarely are willing to accept this assistance. Therefore the management of the hypochondriacal older adult falls primarily on primary care physicians, professionals who work with the elder on a regular basis (such as staff in a nursing home), and the family.

Exaggerated concern about their health is a problem for about 10 percent of older persons. If the more strict criteria for the diagnosis of hypochondriasis is used, the frequency is probably lower, yet no data are available to estimate the frequency of hypochondriasis. A community survey in Durham, North Carolina found that approximately 10 percent of persons 65 years of age and older perceived their physical health to be poorer than it actually was (Blazer and Houpt, 1979). Another 10 percent, however, believed their physical health to be better than determined by objective rating. In another study, 53.6 percent of older adults believed their health to be better than other persons their age. Thirty-one percent felt their health to be about the same as other people their age, whereas only 9.8 percent perceived their health to be poorer than among other older persons (NIDA, 1977).

A more severe form of exaggerated concern about health than hypochondriasis is the so-called somatization disorder, a psychiatric disorder characterized by multiple symptoms that usually begins early in life (often in adolescence). Women are primarily affected and those who suffer hysteria report recurrent, multiple physical problems, which are often described in dramatic fashion. A laundry list of symptoms is reviewed if a clinician inquires, such as difficulty with vision, headaches, stomach pains, constipation, difficulty urinating, and joint pains. These persons repeatedly visit physicians, overuse (and frequently abuse) medication, and receive unnecessary surgery. This severe form of psychosomatic disorder is much less frequent than excessive worry about one's health and afflicts 0.2 to 0.6 percent of older adults in the community.

Both hypochondriasis and somatization disorder are chronic conditions that frustrate health care professionals, which probably contributes to the persistence of the problems. Because older persons can develop real physical problems in the midst of their frequent somatic complaints, they are at higher risk for neglect by their doctors and nurses. In addition, older persons suffering hypochondriasis or somatization disorder may abuse medications or undergo unnecessary and potentially dangerous medical procedures which place them at an increased risk for major medical problems. Although severe consequences resulting from the mental suffering associated with hypochondriasis are less common than for other problems (for example, the risk for suicide is relatively low), the elder may be misdiagnosed as suffering hypochondriasis when in fact a severe depression is manifesting itself with physical symptoms. Major depression characterized by multiple physical problems places an older adult at a higher risk for suicide.

Mrs. Samuels was 73 years old when she appeared for an evaluation in a young physician's office. This young doctor was but the most recent in a long stream of physicians who had been consulted regarding her care. When she arrived at the office, she was accompanied by her son and sister. She was a widow and lived with the sister. Upon entering the examining room, she sighed, "Oh doctor, if you only knew how I've been suffering!" Before the doctor had an opportunity to ask why she had come to the office, she began a tale of woe regarding her physical health that would have taken hours to complete if he had not intervened and structured the interview and examination.

Joint pain was the major complaint, although she also suffered severe pain in her lower back and frequent headaches. Her appetite was poor and she had to "force myself to eat." Food would lodge in her esophagus and she could not swallow. After a meal, she felt an urge to defecate but would find herself severely constipated, which aggravated her hemorrhoids. Suffering from cataracts, her eyesight had been failing for many years. She was waiting for them to "become ripe" so she could receive surgery for the cataracts. Three years prior to the evaluation, she was afflicted by shingles and did not believe she had ever totally recovered from the severe pain she suffered during the infection.

When the doctor discussed Mrs. Samuels' physical problems with her son and sister, no clear date of onset could be established. In fact, since her retirement as a clerk for the state in the Department of Motor Vehicles, she had complained frequently of physical problems. Her son visited her devotedly once a week. He was married to a woman from Germany (whom he had met during military service), however, and yearly returned to Germany for one month so that his wife could visit with her family. Mrs. Samuels' symptoms always became worse prior to his visits abroad. Each year, she feared she would never see him again, given the severity of her medical problems.

Mrs. Samuels' sister vacillated between being a martyr-like caregiver of Mrs. Samuels and an utterly exasperated caregiver. On more than one occasion, the sister had left the house after an argument because all Mrs. Samuels would talk about was her physical health. Though the sister believed Mrs. Samuels could assist with some of the housework, most of it inevitably became her responsibility. After an argument, the sister would return to the home fearing for the physical health of Mrs. Samuels and would encourage her to eat or to take her medications.

Mrs. Samuels had been hospitalized on two occasions for mental problems. The first of these hospitalizations had occurred ten years previously. She suffered at that time severe depressive symptoms and received electroconvulsive therapy (ECT). The depressive symptoms were relieved and she had returned to her work. The second hospitalization had occurred three years previously. During this hospitalization, she also suffered depression, yet the depressive symptoms were more often expressed in physical complaints. The depression did not appear severe enough to warrant ECT and, in fact, the episode was quite different in nature than the one that had responded to ECT. Therefore, her attending physicians prescribed antidepressant medications and tranquilizers along with the multiple medicines she had taken for her various physical problems.

When evaluated by the young doctor, Mrs. Samuels was taking an antidepressant medication (doxepin 10 mg two times a day and 20 mg at night), diazepam (Valium) 2 mg four times a day, flurazepam (Dalmane) 30 mg at bedtime, phenylbutazone (Butazolidin) 100 mg three times a day, and conjugated estrogens (Premarin) 0.25 mg for twenty-one out of every twenty-eight days. She also took Tylenol, an average of four to eight per day.

During the physical examination, the physician elicited some moderate pain on movement of her joints but a full range of motion. Objective abnormalities of the joint were minimal. Blood pressure was normal, her heart sounds were normal and she suffered no neurologic abnormalities. Her mood appeared somewhat discouraged but not depressed. She reported no thoughts of suicide and did not describe any problems in her life (except the occasional arguments with her sister) beyond the physical problems from which she was suffering. Laboratory tests were all normal. Mrs. Samuels is a typical case of hypochondriasis in late life.

Somatoform Disorders

HYPOCHONDRIASIS

Hypochondriasis is classified in our current psychiatric nomenclature under the group of emotional problems known as somatoform disorders, that is, a group of emotional problems dominated by physical symptoms but for which there are no obvious physical findings coupled with a strong assumption that physical symptoms are derived primarily from psychological problems (APA, 1987).

These disorders are to be distinguished from malingering, where the production of symptoms is intentional. The hypochondriac is not aware that the symptoms are the result of an emotional illness.

The most common of the somatoform disorders in late life is hypochondriasis. The essential feature of hypochondriasis is a preoccupation with the fear of having, or the belief that one has, a serious disease, based on the person's interpretation of physical signs or sensations as evidence of physical illness. A thorough history and physical examination do not support the diagnosis of a medical illness that can account for the symptoms and physical signs presented by the older adult. This is not to say that the older person may not suffer some physical disability, but rather that the nature and extent of the physical problems cannot be attributed to that physical illness alone. Despite medical reassurance, the elder suffering hypochondriasis is not relieved of his or her concern. The symptoms, however, do not reach the intensity of a delusion. For example, the hypochondriacal elder does not complain, "I know I have a cancer. It is just that they have not found that cancer yet." Rather, the elder complains, "I just feel certain something is wrong with me, but the doctors can't seem to find anything. They tend to dismiss the suffering I'm experiencing. Maybe they are right, but nothing they've suggested makes the pain go away."

Hypochondriacal symptoms last for at least six months (in order to meet criteria for the diagnosis) and the elder suffering the disorder becomes increasingly preoccupied with body functioning. Any perceived change in heartbeat, sensation to heat or cold, bowel cramps, a new cough, or the development of a new pain heightens the anxiety related to hypochondriasis.

Fear of having a disease that is unrecognized or neglected leads the elderly hypochondriac to doctor shop. As Mrs. Samuels exhibited, these patients move from one doctor to another in search of an answer to their problems. They also tend to retain the services of multiple medical specialists simultaneously, such as an ophthalmologist, an internist, and a rheumatologist as well as a primary care physician. Hypochondriasis can be seen in both men and women. Although the onset usually occurs between 20 and 30 years of age, hypochondriasis tends to become more severe in mid-life and persists into late life. Persons suffering hypochondriasis generally maintain a relatively productive life, but occupational functioning is often undermined and the elderly hypochondriac frequently retires early for health reasons. The preoccupation of the elder with physical problems, as exhibited by Mrs. Samuels, often strains social relations.

The elder suffering from hypochondriasis, that is, the elder who presents multiple, unexplained complaints to a professional, must not be neglected by health care professionals. Not only may an older adult develop a physical illness in the midst of multiple unexplained physical symptoms, some medical problems are not easily diagnosed initially. Multiple sclerosis often begins with a series of unexplained and frequently ignored physical complaints, only to manifest itself as a severe neurologic disorder later in the course of the disorder. Thyroid disorders or hyperactivity of the adrenal gland (Cushing's disease), as well as diseases that affect multiple body symptoms such as systemic lupus erythematosus (SLE), may not be easily identified early in their course.

SOMATIZATION DISORDER

As noted above, a more severe somatoform disorder is *somatization disorder*. As with hypochondriasis, the essential feature of this disorder is the recurrent and multiple complaints of physical problems, lasting several years, for which medical attention has been frequently sought. No physical disorder can be identified to explain the symptoms.

As with hypochondriasis, the somatization disorder begins earlier in life and has a chronic but fluctuating course. The severity of the problem, however, is greater than hypochondriasis. To qualify for a diagnosis of somatization disorder, the elder must suffer at least thirteen physical symptoms that are not explained by physical illness, the use of a medication, or alcohol. They may complain of such symptoms as gastrointestinal problems, such as vomiting, abdominal pain, nausea, and diarrhea; unexplained pains, such as back pain, joint pain, and pain on urination; symptoms of heart and lung dysfunction, such as shortness of breath without exertion, pounding of the heart, chest pains, and dizziness; neurologic or conversion symptoms, such as amnesia, difficulty swallowing, loss of voice, blurred vision, and difficulty walking; symptoms of sexual dysfunction, such as burning of the sexual organs, pain during intercourse, and impotence; and symptoms of the female reproductive system, such as excessive menstrual bleeding, irregular menstrual periods, and painful menstruation.

Unlike hypochondriasis, somatization disorder is much more common in females than in males, and, as noted above, the frequency of the disorder is lower than for hypochondriasis. Some suggest that the disorder is in part hereditary and associated with antisocial personality disorder or drug abuse in males. That is, in the families where somatization disorder is common among females, males suffer drug and alcohol abuse as well as antisocial personality disorder.

The extremes to which persons suffering somatization disorder go in order to obtain medical attention exceed those for hypochondriasis. These persons are constantly consulting doctors and doctor shop even more frequently than persons suffering hypochondriasis. They not uncommonly are hospitalized and undergo exploratory surgery, x rays, a myriad of laboratory tests, and a trial on many medications. Exploratory abdominal, rectal, and gallbladder surgery are common. These patients may be hospitalized scores of times during their life and frequently are hospitalized on psychiatric wards as well as medical and surgery wards. Hypochondriacal patients, in contrast, are rarely hospitalized on psychiatric services (Mrs. Samuels was an exception).

SOMATOFORM PAIN DISORDER

The third condition included among the somatoform disorders affecting older adults is the *somatoform pain disorder*. The central feature of this problem is preoccupation with pain in the absence of adequate physical findings to account for the pain or its intensity. Unlike hypochondriasis and somatization disorder, the complaint in somatoform pain disorder is localized to one area of the body, especially the back. To qualify for the diagnosis, the pain must have lasted for at least six months. Medical evaluation often uncovers no physical problem to explain the pain. If the elder does suffer a physical problem (such as ruptured disc), the nature and extent of the pain or the resulting social and occupational impairment is much greater than what would be expected from the physical problem alone (APA, 1987). Somatoform pain disorder is more prevalent in mid-life than in late life but is relatively common throughout life. Onset of the somatoform pain disorder is usually sudden (often associated with an injury) and tends to increase in severity over the first weeks and months following the injury. The problem, like hypochondriasis and somatization disorder, often persists for many years. Rarely does the pain disappear once it has been present over a year.

The Etiology of Hypochondriasis

By definition, little biologic cause can be identified for hypochondriasis. Therefore, once physical illness has been ruled out as primarily responsible for the problem, the clinician must look for psychological and psychosocial causes. Busse (1989) suggested four mechanisms that contribute to hypochondriasis in the elderly. First, symptoms may be used to explain failure to meet personal or social expectations and to avoid or excuse recurrent failure. Older adults do not commonly face as many challenges, such as filling social roles, as persons in mid-life and usually are not faced with the necessity to compete: nevertheless, certain expectations are placed upon elders. Failure to meet these expectations can greatly damage self-esteem. For example, a child may ask his grandfather to throw a baseball. The child has played with his father and admired him for his athletic abilities. Possibly grandfather was an excellent athlete during high school or college days (something described to the grandchild by the child's parents). Nevertheless, skills have been lost and the elder may fear embarrassing himself in the situation. Therefore, the older man complains of pain in the back, arthritic pains in the shoulder, or exhaustion to excuse exposing inadequacy in physical sports.

Second, the older adult may experience increased isolation and respond to this isolation by withdrawing interest in those around and focusing that interest on himself or herself, especially the body and its functions. When the elder does not receive a phone call, tires of television, and finds little to do around the house after routine chores have been completed, the body can become a focus of concern. Body functions are continually in process and can easily attract attention when there is little to displace that attention from the social surroundings. Most persons can sit for a few moments perfectly still with eyes closed in a quiet room and begin to feel physical discomfort if not allowed to fall asleep. By adjusting their position in a chair or moving they might overcome this discomfort. The elder begins to attend to bowel movements, color of the skin, changes in vision, aches from every joint, brief episodes of dizziness, acceleration of the heartbeat, or changes in response to the ambient temperature. When social contact does occur, the elder immediately wishes to share what has occupied his mind during the previous hours (or even days), that is, the body.

A third mechanism that predisposes to hypochondriacal symptoms is an attempt by the older adult to shift anxiety from specific psychological conflicts to a less threatening problem with a bodily function. The older adult, for example, may fear the loss of memory. Someone who has valued his or her mind for many years (such as a college professor or an engineer) may be extremely threatened by the possibility of a diminishing clarity of thinking and memory. If memory is challenged, anxiety increases. One means of alleviating this anxiety is to focus on bodily symptoms and therefore ignore the memory loss. If the elder is preoccupied with a pain in the stomach, how will he or she have time to concentrate upon problems with memory?

The fourth of the mechanisms described by Busse is the use of hypochondriacal symptoms to punish oneself or to provide some type of atonement for unacceptable hostile feelings felt toward another person. When an older couple retires, they begin to spend much more time together than they have previously. Such increased time not infrequently leads to increased tension within the marriage. Nevertheless, the expression of such hostility and the unexpressed wish to have the husband or wife "out of the house" may not be acceptable, given the culture in which the older person resides. Therefore, the elder chooses instead to redirect these hostile feelings toward the self. "If I wish my wife were out of the house and do not care for her after these many years, I'm a bad person. If I'm bad I should be punished. Possibly this pain that I feel in my back and the weakness I experience are a way for me to be punished." If the older person does not consciously follow this line of reasoning to self-punishment, nevertheless, the subconscious dynamics of managing the feelings of hostility can end with the hostility directed toward the self and then toward the body.

Psychoanalysts have recognized that such psychological defense mechanisms, as described, are not the only force driving the appearance and persistence of hypochondriacal symptoms. Once a symptom emerges, much so-called secondary gain may derive from the symptom. Friends and relatives direct increased attention to the older adult who expresses multiple physical problems. Professionals working with older adults must recognize the secondary gain, for even the best therapeutic plans are doomed to failure if it is not understood. The older adult has an investment in retaining the symptoms and therefore, subconsciously, will undermine attempts to alleviate the pain and suffering.

Another equally important mechanism that may lead to persistent hypochondriasis is a persistent depressive disorder. Lesse (1974) notes that depressive symptoms may be hidden for long periods of time by hypochondriacal symptoms. Such patients, suffering a chronic depression, engage clinicians in long, circumstantial discussions of their problems. At the end of the interview, however, the clinician remains confused regarding the nature, extent and functional impairment suffered by the older adult. Depressed hypochondriacal patients, in contrast to other hypochondriacs, emphasize repeatedly the great suffering that they have endured. Social and job-related performance is more likely to be impaired in the depressed elder. In addition to the usual bodily complaints, the depressed elder emphasizes the tension and anxiety associated with the symptoms as well as insomnia, loss of appetite, and fatigue (often with the problems being experienced more in the mornings than in the afternoons). Poor memory and difficulty concentrating are prominent symptoms in depression as well. Nevertheless, these patients repeatedly refer back to their physical illness. Hopelessness as evidenced by statements such as "I know I'm never going to get any better" are characteristic of the depressed hypochondriac. Suicidal thoughts are not uncommon and suicide is a risk for such individuals. The depressed elder who focuses upon his or her physical problems appears to suffer more than the hypochondriacal elder.

Social factors also contribute to hypochondriacal symptoms. In addition to the secondary gain derived from the symptoms, as described above, the older person expressing hypochondriacal problems is able to assume the "sick role." The sick in our society fill a special role. Not only are they not expected to maintain gainful employment, attend school, or meet other usual social obligations, they can, with impunity, depend on others. They are not expected to care for themselves, require continuing medical attention, and can discharge social responsibilities to others (such as the responsibility of managing one's finances). The more severe the perceived illness, the more likely is the older adult to be treated as dependent (Atchley, 1985).

The Diagnostic Workup

The office evaluation of the hypochondriacal older adult is founded upon a thorough history, including the careful evaluation of former medical problems (which includes the voluminous records that have accumulated). Time spent early in the diagnostic process to formulate a comprehensive picture of the medical, psychological, and social aspects of the physical complaints is time well spent (Blazer, 1984). The diagnostic workup—including the history, physical examination, mental status examination, and laboratory tests—should not only assist the clinician in distinguishing symptoms of predominant psychological derivation from true physical illness but also enable the clinician to distinguish hypochondriasis from other psychiatric problems.

EVALUATION OF THE HYPOCHONDRIACAL ELDER

In the history-taking process, the clinician should first focus upon the symptoms of most concern to the suffering elder and the duration of these symptoms as well as their changing pattern over time. Are the symptoms episodic or have they persisted unchanged for months or even years? Past history of medical illness (with a focus upon a review of past hospitalizations and use of medications) clarifies the subjective report by the older adult. Past psychiatric history should be elicited as well, for some of these elders, though they do not report emotional problems nor do they attribute their problems to emotional causes, nevertheless, have received psychiatric care, even hospital care. A thorough medication history is essential, including those medications that are taken at present, both on a regular and on an as-needed basis. Interviews with the family can assist in documenting the accuracy of reports of medication use and daily function. To what extent does the hypochondriacal elder continue functioning? For example, attendance at religious activities, visits with the family, shopping trips, and other usual activities should be explored. If these have been greatly limited, then an evaluation of functional capacity (activities of daily living) is essential.

A thorough evaluation of activities of daily living generally focuses upon both instrumental activities of living and self-care capacity. Instrumental activities include those activities that are instrumental in permitting the older adult to maintain independent function in the community. The ability to cook one's meals, shop, use the telephone, pay the bills, and the like, should be reviewed. Next the older person should be questioned as to his or her ability to bathe, dress, groom (brush one's teeth, comb one's hair, and so on), feed oneself and move around within the home.

Self-report of activities of daily living by the hypochondriacal older adult is not as accurate as might be desired. For this reason, the clinician can ask the older person to perform certain tasks (such as moving from a sitting to a standing position, holding a semi-heavy object for 20 to 30 seconds, and writing one's name) in order to verify capabilities. Family members should also be asked about the capacity and the actual performance of these activities by the hypochondriacal elder.

The physical examination during the first visit should be as complete as possible. Blood pressure, pulse, range of motion of the extremities, evaluation of the lungs and heart, and a careful examination of the skin are essential. A rectal examination should be performed, as well as a stool analysis for blood (guaiac test). The neurologic examination is very important, though again the results may be less than accurate due to lack of cooperation by the hypochondriacal elder (either conscious or unconscious).

During the mental status examination, it is essential to encourage the older adult to perform as well as possible, especially on cognitive testing. Mood should be assessed both in terms of self-report on the degree of suffering or discomfort and an evaluation by the clinician as to the degree of suffering by the older person. The presence of suicidal thoughts is important to document. Clinicians can expect continued somatic complaints throughout the mental status examination but should persist through the exam until it is completed.

The clinician does not usually expect any abnormalities on laboratory testing. Nevertheless, if the clinician is evaluating the hypochondriacal elder for the first time, routine laboratory testing is essential. An automated blood count and differential as well as a urinalysis and a chemical screen are most helpful. If thyroid function tests and liver function tests have not been performed in the recent past, they should be obtained as well. The same is true for the chest x ray and electrocardiogram. Careful completion of the diagnostic workup, even if it requires multiple office visits, will eventually save the clinician from unnecessary repeats of tests and added time during the ensuing period of care.

As mentioned above, one of the important tasks during the diagnostic process is to distinguish hypochondriacal patients from patients suffering other psychiatric disorders. Depressive disorders can be distinguished from hypochondriasis through a number of characteristics. In general, patients suffering depressive disorders appear to "suffer" their symptoms much more than the hypochondriacal patient, although depressive disorders can lead to hypochondriasis. Hostility in the hypochondriacal patient is usually directed outward, though hypochondriasis may result from inward directed hostility. A much more likely cause for anger directed inward is a depressive disorder. Social withdrawal tends to be more prominent with the depressive disorders. Chronicity is more likely to reflect hypochondriasis than depression. Depressive disorders also tend to be more cyclic (with remissions and relapses) than hypochondriasis. The hypochondriacal patient is less willing to discuss psychological problems and social difficulties, even with coaxing, than the depressed patient. Even during therapy, some differences emerge. The hypochondriacal patient generally will not tolerate the side effects of the more commonly used psychotherapeutic drugs, especially the antidepressant medications (Blazer, 1984).

Hypochondriasis can be distinguished from organic brain disorders as follows: The somatic concern among the demented tends to be episodic, whereas the somatic concern of the hypochondriacal patient is persistent. Both conditions, however, are chronic. A hypochondriacal elder and a demented elder both perform poorly on the mental status examination, but the results are more varied for the hypochondriacal patient when the test is repeated than for the demented patient. Anxiety generally increases during the mental status examination in the demented patient, whereas the examination rarely produces anxiety in the hypochondriacal patient. The demented patient generally shows deterioration through time, whereas the hypochondriacal patient rarely exhibits such deterioration (Blazer, 1984).

EVALUATION OF THE FAMILY

Evaluation of the family is an essential step in the diagnostic workup of the hypochondriacal older adult. Unwillingness to perform usual daily activities or even neglect of personal hygiene coupled with repeated vocalization of needs places a burden on family members (Blazer, 1984). The subsequent relationship within the family is one of both dependence and hostility. Hypochondriacal behavior itself may send a message to family members, suggesting "you have caused me to feel so bad. Can't you see how little you care?" Family members, though they may not recognize the message consciously, respond subconsciously with both guilt and anger. This in turn may lead to the vicious cycle of family members reinforcing the hypochondriacal elder's suffering and dependence.

On occasion, more than one family member may suffer hypochondriasis. Although spouses rarely experience hypochondriasis simultaneously, when two elderly siblings live together, there may be considerable competition for attention and hostility expressed, representing sibling rivalries of many years duration. Who has the most problems? Who deserves the most attention? Whose turn is it to receive attention from the other sibling or family? Occasionally, hypochondriasis may arise when another family member is suffering a serious physical or emotional illness.

A further component of the evaluation of the hypochondriacal elder's family is the assessment of the perceived ability of the family to respond to and care for the needs of the hypochondriacal elder versus the actual capabilities of the family to provide such care. Patterns of interaction within stressed families tend to be conflictual and the family as a unit does not function well, thus leading to difficulty in responding to the continual demands of the hypochondriacal elder (Blazer, 1984). At times, families will respond excessively, lavishing much care on the dependent and demanding elder. At other times, frustration with the repeated demands leads to withdrawal of family members, if not abuse and abandonment of their elder. Even in the midst of a true crisis, such families can be slow to respond. The clinician must evaluate the capability of the family to respond to an emergency, as well as catalogue the tangible supports provided to the elder, such as transportation, meal preparation, supervision (especially supervision of medications) and financial assistance (such as a realistic appraisal of resources of medical care). In families with a dependent elder, the clinician can usually identify a "manager" who is somewhat distant to the day-to-day conflicts within the family and is in the best position to provide the most logical assessment of family needs and to garner the resources necessary to meet those needs. When the clinician can identify this manager, successful intervention is more likely (see Chapter 12).

Treatment of the Hypochondriacal Elder

Because there is little biologic basis for the symptoms of hypochondriasis, the treatment is primarily directed to the psychological and social dysfunction associated with the problem. Treatment for both hypochondriasis and somatization disorder is similar (and therefore will be discussed together). The treatment of the somatoform pain disorder is somewhat different but will not be discussed here, as the problem is less frequent in later life. The use of medication may, at times, be indicated in the treatment of hypochondriasis and somatization disorder. Nevertheless, medication must be placed within the context of a consistent psychosocial approach to treatment. Therefore, pharmacologic therapy for hypochondriasis and somatization disorder will be discussed within this context.

Busse (1954) suggested a series of guidelines for treating the hypochondriacal patient. First, the clinician must recognize that the patient is "ill." Making such comments as "It's all in your mind" or "Don't worry about this pain" only fuels the fire of the symptoms presented to the clinician. Persons can suffer from an illness without the clinician being able to identify the exact cause of the illness or being able to respond to a specific therapy. Anyone suffering a physical illness, real or imagined, deserves the attention of a professional. Next, the clinician should commit himself or herself to the assistance of the patient. Statements such as "I don't know exactly the cause of your problem, and I'm not certain that I can provide immediate relief. Nevertheless, I will work with you as best I can to find a solution," are most encouraging to the hypochondriacal elder.

Such commitment does not imply that unreasonable amounts of time or the prescription of inappropriate therapies is necessary. Commitment, at times, is best expressed to the elder by careful attention to the symptoms at the first visit.

Once the initial evaluation has been completed, return visits should be structured (for structure is the key to effective management of the hypochondriacal patient). The goal is to control the suffering of the patient as well as the use of health services by these patients. Clinicians should agree to see the patient on a regular basis, frequently at first and then spaced out with time. During each visit, a set amount of time should be allotted to the elder (about twenty minutes). A brief interval history is obtained from the patient and an even briefer physical examination (usually requiring about five minutes and including blood pressure determination, heart rate monitoring, and listening to the chest and heart) should be performed. During the remainder of the visit, patients should, within a relaxed atmosphere, be encouraged to discuss personal and social concerns. An expression of interest in these concerns, without suggesting that these psychosocial problems are the cause of the physical symptoms, provides an atmosphere that encourages the elder to ventilate those problems of concern. Many elders suffering hypochondriasis believe that if they talk about personal problems to a clinician, then the clinician will deemphasize or at least not believe that the elder is suffering a physical problem (the only legitimate reason that the elder can seek medical care). Given the propensity of hypochondriacal patients to use medical services excessively, twenty minutes twelve or fifteen times a year in a primary care physician's office discussing emotional problems is a most cost-efficient means of caring for the hypochondriacal patient.

Emphasis on a predetermined amount of time for each visit is essential in the care of the hypochondriacal patient. The consultation should be begun and terminated promptly, even if the patient appears to leave the most important issues to the last minute. Statements such as "This appears to be a very important topic, but our time is up today and we can talk about that during our next visit," can be used to terminate the session. The clinician should avoid retaliation or arguments with the patient about both current and past medical care. Rather, clear statements should be made regarding the physician's judgment as to the relative benefit versus danger of given medications, continually emphasizing that the overall well-being of the patient is the prime concern.

Once a therapeutic relationship is established, hypochondriacal patients often wish to discuss bad experiences they have encountered with other clinicians. The current clinician should avoid defending or criticizing these physicians. Active interest in the concerns and feelings of the hypochondriacal patient is the key ingredient in effective care. Referrals should be kept to a minimum. Hypochondriacal patients, as illustrated by Mrs. Samuels, tend to use many different physicians, thus complicating a consistent approach to care. These patients are best cared for by primary care physicians who only refer when a new symptom emerges that cannot be explained on the basis of knowledge about the patient's overall condition.

It is difficult to care for a hypochondriacal patient without prescribing some medication. The use of a placebo (a sugar pill) is unwarranted for it may destroy the clinician-patient relationship. Physicians should be honest with patients about what they are prescribing at all times. Nevertheless, medications can be prescribed that have few side effects and are of value for symptomatic relief. Prescription of such medications can control the elder's shopping for a doctor or collecting a pharmacy in the medicine cabinet at home. For example, L-tryptophan can be prescribed for difficulty in sleeping (the drug can be prescribed or bought over the counter). Two grams of L-tryptophan have virtually no side effects (though a recent scare regarding the drug emerged, probably because one batch of the medication was improperly processed). The drug at that dose is mildly sedating. Diphenhydramine (Benadryl) is available over the counter in 25 or 50 mg doses, and may cause drowsiness. Benadryl, however, is not a sedative/hypnotic as is flurazepam (Dalmane). The ability of Dalmane to induce and maintain sleep far exceeds Benadryl. Yet the clinician does not need to be concerned about habituation with Benadryl. Benadryl can cause side effects (such as blurring of vision, constipation, or even confusion) and must be monitored carefully. Analgesics such as acetaminophen or ibuprofen can be prescribed as well. At times, hypochondriacal patients do not believe they have value from a visit to a physician's office if they do not leave the office with a prescription.

The goals of treating the hypochondriacal elder must be kept in view if the day-to-day difficulties in managing these patients are to be overcome. "Treatment" is misleading, for the major goal is management and control (Blazer, 1984). Even though specific hypochondriacal symptoms occasionally remit, the disorder is chronic. Management goals include:

1. Decrease and control the use of health care services.
2. Decrease the concern and anxiety of the hypochondriacal elder concerning the availability and commitment of health care professionals.
3. Decrease stress on the family.
4. Increase the capabilities of the family to provide a supportive environment to the hypochondriacal elder (though not an environment that supports continued dependence).
5. Decrease conflict within the family.
6. Decrease anxiety within the patient.

There are a number of therapies by which the management of the hypochondriacal patient can be expanded beyond the office of the primary care physician. These therapies are relatively cost-efficient and can provide considerable support for hypochondriacal elders. They include biofeedback, physical therapy, exercise programs, and nutritional programs. Physical therapy is especially valuable to hypochondriacal elders who are inpatients and can be extended to the home once the patient is discharged. A concerned physical therapist who works carefully with the older person thirty minutes three to four times a week provides much needed support to the symptom-burdened elder.

There is a need for working with the family of the hypochondriacal patient as well, based on the evaluation obtained during the diagnostic assessment. Some goals for family (or psychosocial) intervention include (Blazer, 1984):

1. Interview family members for a brief period (if possible) on a regular basis while the patient is being evaluated. Although family members should be interviewed each time the elder sees the clinician, family interviews can be decreased with time.

2. Do not relate to the family that the problem is primarily or solely an emotional one (thus increasing the hostility between the family and the hypochondriacal elder).
3. The clinician, if possible, should avoid treating more than one patient who has excessive physical problems within a given family. Multiple hypochondriacs seeking attention from a busy clinician engender competition between family members for the attention of the clinician.
4. The family should be assured that adequate medical care will be provided to the patient (to ease those times when the elder pressures family that he is not receiving adequate medical attention and cries for another evaluation).
5. Assure the family that the hypochondriacal symptoms, though chronic, are not life-threatening. Nevertheless, the family should recognize that the hypochondriacal elder can become seriously ill at any time, despite the best of medical attention.
6. Be certain that the hypochondriacal elder and other family members are not "sharing medications." A major goal of therapy with the family is to control the use of medications. It is essential for the clinician to assess and instruct family members to not allow the hypochondriacal elder to use medicines that may be available in the home (that is, medications prescribed for other family members).
7. The clinician should always maintain a neutral position, avoiding "taking sides" with family members against a patient or with the patient against the family members.
8. The clinician should encourage the family to support the patient's attempts to become more independent. In addition, the clinician should encourage the caregivers to seek respite, for daily care of the hypochondriacal elder can be exhausting.

References

American Psychological Association. *Diagnostic and Statistical Manual of Mental Disorders* (3d ed.). Washington, DC: American Psychological Association, 1987.

Atchley, R. C. *Social Forces and Aging.* Belmont, CA: Wadsworth, 1985.

Blazer, D. G. "Hypochondriasis." In D. G. Blazer and I. C. Siegler (Eds.), *A Family Approach to Health Care in the Elderly.* Menlo Park, CA: Addison-Wesley Publishing Co., 1984. Pp. 140–156.

Blazer, D. G., and J. L. Houpt. "Perception of poor health in the healthy older adult." *Journal of the American Geriatric Society*, 27:330, 1979.

Busse, E. W. "The treatment of hypochondriasis." *Tri-State Medical Journal*, 2:7, 1954.

Busse, E. W. "Somatoform and psychosocial disorders." In E. W. Busse and D. G. Blazer (Eds.), *Geriatric Psychiatry.* Washington, DC: American Psychiatric Press, 1989. Pp. 429–458.

Lesse, S. "Hypochondriasis and psychosomatic disorders." In S. Lesse (Ed.), *Masked Depression.* New York: Jason Aronson, 1974. Pp. 53–74.

NIDA Services Research Report. *A Study of Legal Drug Use by Older Americans.* DHEW Publication 77-495. Washington, DC: Department of Health, Education, and Welfare, 1977.

Suggested Reading

Barsky, A., and G. L. Klerman. "Overview of hypochondriasis: Bodily complaint and somatic styles." *American Journal of Psychiatry*, 140:273, 1983.

Ford, C. V. *The Somatosizing Disorders.* New York: Elsevier, 1983.

Viderman, M. "Somatoform and factitious disorders." In R. Michaels and J. O. Cavenar (Eds.), *Psychiatry*, Volume 1. Philadelphia: J. B. Lippincott, 1987.

CHAPTER EIGHT

Sleeping Problems

Sigmund Freud (1917), in his introductory lectures on psychoanalysis, noted, "The world, it seems, does not possess even those of us who are adults completely, but only up to two thirds; one third of us is still quite unborn. Every time we awake in the morning it is like a new birth." Most persons scarcely give sleep a second thought, however, until they encounter problems with their sleep. Few symptoms can lead to more discomfort and frustration than difficulty with sleep.

Insomnia increases proportionally with age (Lugaresi et al., 1987). Over the age of 80, nearly 50 percent of persons surveyed complained of difficulty with their sleep. In a review of the literature on sleep, Dement et al., (1982) found 15 percent of persons over 65 slept fewer than five hours a night, with sleep complaints reported twice as frequently among females compared to males. About 25 to 30 percent of both men and women reported frequent night awakenings with 15 percent reporting that they awoke early in the morning (usually before 5 A.M.). One quarter of the men over the age of 65 and 40 percent of the women described their sleep as light. Nearly 10 percent of the elderly reported using sleeping pills at least part of the time. A case of sleeping problems is presented below.

Mr. Franklin had trained horses most of his adult life. He operated three stables and had been most successful in this business. Five years prior to seeing a psychiatrist, he turned the business over to his two daughters. Following that transition, he found himself with little to do and concurrently began to argue with his daughters regarding their methods of operating the stables and riding academy.

It was not problems with his daughters, however, that brought Mr. Franklin to the psychiatrist's office at least once a month. Rather, he complained of difficulty sleeping. The psychiatrist had tried numerous medications and finally referred him to a sleep specialist to evaluate the sleep problem. When he reported to the specialist Mr. Franklin was taking 50 mg of Benadryl (diphenhydramine) and 30 mg of Dalmane (flurazepam), and he would repeat the Dalmane at least once during the night. He usually began his ritual of trying to get a good night's sleep around 10:00 P.M. After a warm bath and a glass of warm milk, he would take the Dalmane and Benadryl and turn off the lights. Most nights, however, he found that he was not sleepy. He would get up at least once or twice, wander to the kitchen or turn on the television, only to become drowsy, and return to the bed. Finally, he would fall asleep.

Three to four hours into the night, Mr. Franklin usually awakened, needing to urinate. After urinating he would return to bed and once again could not fall asleep. If he remained awake more than thirty minutes, he would take the second Dalmane (about five nights out of seven). He would look at his digital clock frequently and knew exactly the times that he awakened and how long he remained awake during the night.

After the second Dalmane, Mr. Franklin would again fall asleep for a couple of hours, only to awaken around 4:00 to 4:30 A.M. When he awoke that early, he became frustrated, believing that he had not received enough sleep during the night, and would attempt to "nap" until 6:00 in the morning. This napping was light, and he experienced short dreams that excited or disturbed him. Upon arising in the morning, he would feel both tired and anxious. After drinking a cup of coffee and reading the paper he would each day take a walk for about an hour and the walk calmed him. After the walk, his wife would awaken and they would eat breakfast.

As the afternoon approached, Mr. Franklin became drowsy and would take a nap. This nap would usually last 1 to 1½ hours, and Mr. Franklin never felt especially rested afterward. Upon awakening, he felt relatively well the remainder of the day. During the evening, he felt better than any other time of day. As 9:00 approached, however, his anxiety would increase as he would anticipate the problems he would have in sleeping that night.

During the evaluation, the sleep specialist identified no other problems with Mr. Franklin except the sleep difficulties. A sleep study (see below) was ordered. Although it was suspected the sleep study would be less than adequate given that Mr. Franklin refused to stop taking his sleeping pills for even one night, as he dreaded the possibility of an entire night without sleep. (Sleep studies, if used to document the natural physiologic patterns of sleep, should be performed in a natural state, that is, without medications.) The sleep study revealed that Mr. Franklin slept a total of 4½ hours during the night. For him, it required thirty minutes after the lights were turned off to enter stage 1 sleep (see below) and he awakened six or seven times during the night, only to return to sleep five to fifteen minutes afterwards. He would awaken for the last time around 5:00 in the morning.

The sleep specialist suggested that Mr. Franklin enter a hospital and be withdrawn from the sleep medications, as they were suspected to be contributing to his sleep problems. He reluctantly agreed. Over a ten-day period, the Benadryl and the Dalmane were gradually withdrawn. His sleep, during the withdrawal period, initially became worse, but then about five or six days after the drugs had been withdrawn, his sleep improved. He was cautioned that he should avoid sleeping pills in the future.

Instead, a program of good sleep hygiene was instituted. Mr. Franklin was instructed to continue to drink the warm milk and take the warm shower before bedtime. He was cautioned, however, not to exercise after 5:00 P.M. (in order that he may not become overly activated in the evenings). The face of the digital clock was turned away from the bed (so he could not monitor the time during which he slept during the night). He obtained a white noise machine, which he used during the winter (substituting a fan during the summer). The bedroom was kept at a constant temperature (about 68°). Mr. Franklin was encouraged to get up and read a book (rather than watching television) if he could not sleep. As he became bored quickly with reading and subsequently drowsy, he rarely remained up more than five or ten minutes before returning to bed. He was encouraged to not nap more than thirty minutes a day, using an alarm clock to awaken him from the nap.

Mr. Franklin faithfully followed this program of sleep hygiene and reported that his sleep was somewhat better, though he continued to worry about his sleep. A repeat sleep study was performed. During this study, it was found that Mr. Franklin was sleeping a total of 6½ hours at night. The time between turning the lights out and falling asleep was *decreased from thirty to ten minutes. When he awakened to urinate around 2:00 A.M., Mr. Franklin was able to return to bed and to fall asleep in approximately ten minutes. He felt more rested in the mornings and, with encouragement, was able to refrain from further use of sleep medications. With time, he worried less about his sleep, though he rarely got what he considered to be a "good night's sleep."*

Sleep Disorders

Mr. Franklin suffered from insomnia frequently seen among the elderly. *Insomnia* is classified in the psychiatric nomenclature (APA, 1987) as one of the dyssomnias—a disturbance in the amount, quality, or timing of sleep. The major complaint is difficulty in initiating and maintaining sleep or a complaint that sleep does not restore energy and leaves the person tired during the day.

Hypersomnia, or excessive daytime sleepiness or prolonged periods of sleep, is uncommon in late life. Taking naps, however, is a common practice among elders. Problems with the sleep-wake schedule are a major concern for older adults (as exemplified in part by Mr. Franklin's story).

Two types of *sleep-wake schedule disorders* are recognized by professionals. The central feature of sleep-wake disorders is an uncoupling of the normal sleep-wake schedule that is demanded by the person's environment and the person's internal biologic (circadian) rhythm. Complaints of a sleep-wake disorder include insomnia, inability to sleep, and inability to remain alert when wakefulness is necessary (APA, 1987). In *advanced sleep-wake disorder*, the older adult shifts the period of sleep. For example, he or she may go to bed at 6:00 or 7:00 P.M. only to awaken at 2:00 or 3:00 A.M. In *delayed sleep-wake disorder*, the older person does not fall asleep until 2:00 or 3:00 A.M. and awakens late in the morning, around 11:00 A.M. Medication can mask a delayed or advanced sleep-wake disorder. In those cases, elders feel drowsy and do not function well during the period they should be sleeping, given their circadian rhythm. They sleep on medications when they normally should be awake. Advanced and delayed sleep disorders occur frequently in persons who are travelling between time zones. As older adults are less likely to be constrained by schedules, they are especially at risk for developing sleep-wake schedule problems.

The third type is the *disorganized sleep disorder*. Persons with this disorder experience a random pattern of sleep and wake with no regular daily major sleep pattern. Elders who do not follow a schedule may sleep haphazardly and snatch moments of sleep throughout the day and night. People who are bedridden are especially prone to the disorganized type of sleep-wake disorder.

Other problems experienced by older adults during sleep include sleep apnea and sleep-related periodic leg movements. *Sleep apnea*—episodes in which breathing stops for a few seconds during sleep—are common in the elderly and increase with age. One study of older adults found sleep apneas in 24 percent of a sample of community resident seniors (Mosko et al., 1988). Sleep apnea can cause excessive daytime drowsiness, and it disrupts nighttime sleep, although the elder is often unaware that he or she has not slept fitfully. Elders with sleep apnea do complain of not feeling rested in the morning.

How dangerous are these apneas? Most of these apneic episodes lower oxygen levels less than 5 percent, because breathing returns as a reaction to even minimal decreases in oxygen. Heart rate increases less than ten beats per minute. When breathing stops, greater pressure is placed on the heart to deliver oxygen to the remainder of the body. One type of sleep apnea appears to be attributable to a "central mechanism"; the person stops breathing because the respiratory center in the brain briefly ceases to function. Another type of apnea is obstructive; the soft tissue in the pharynx and throat relaxes to the point that the soft tissue obstructs the flow of air into the lungs. Obstructive sleep apnea is therefore associated with an increased frequency of snoring.

Sleep apneas become severe when the elder experiences multiple episodes of apnea through the night and the episodes are of longer duration. Sleep can be interrupted hundreds of times a night in some victims. In most cases, the sleeper is unaware of the repeated awakenings caused by the apnea. He only experiences lethargy and tiredness the next day. The condition can be especially dangerous, in that prolonged apneic episodes can precipitate rhythm problems of the heart and can increase blood pressure (which places the older adult at greater risk for a heart attack) and difficulty with mental processes.

Another sleep problem afflicting many older persons is *periodic leg movements*. Though not as life-threatening as the sleep apneas, these leg movements can be more disturbing, and elders complain of them frequently to their clinicians. The elder experiences a slight twitching of the legs during sleep. These usually occur early in the night during the light stages of sleep (stage 1 or 2). The movements may continue for a few minutes or a few hours. The movements are uncomfortable and usually arouse the elder when he or she is near falling asleep. The elder may be so uncomfortable that he or she gets out of bed and walks around in order to decrease the uncomfortable sensation. If the elder is awakened by the movements many times during the night, he or she is deprived of the deeper stages of sleep and experiences excessive daytime sleepiness, lethargy, and difficulty functioning during the day. As many as 15 percent of the general population (and probably a higher percentage of older adults) complain of periodic leg movements.

A number of drugs increase the likelihood of the periodic leg movements. These drugs include the benzodiazepine drugs (such as Dalmane or Valium), antidepressant medications (such as Pamelor and the MAO inhibitors), caffeine, and alcohol. Some medications have been recommended for the restless leg syndrome and periodic movements of sleep. Clinicians report only modest therapeutic success for any of these agents. One milligram of clonazepam before bedtime does relieve the discomfort in some situations, as does L-tryptophan.

The Etiology of Insomnia or Sleep Abnormalities

THE BIOLOGY OF SLEEP

To understand the causes of sleep abnormalities, it is necessary to review the biology of sleep. Sleep is not a single state (as contrasted to wakefulness), but it is a mixture of several states or stages (Marsh et al., 1987). The stages of sleep are repeated throughout the night. Upon going to bed and turning out the lights, elders first relax their minds and enter a stage known to persons who practice meditation—alpha rhythms. Alpha rhythms designate the background frequency of electrical impulses from the brain recorded by an electroencephalographic tracing (an EEG). The alpha rhythm is a frequency from 8 to 12 cycles per second.

From alpha rhythm, the older adult enters stage 1 sleep. Alpha rhythm gradually disappears and the background activity slows to seven or less cycles per second (theta waves). After fifteen to twenty minutes, stage 1 sleep gradually disappears and the elder enters an even deeper sleep characterized by slower waves and increased voltage (stage 2 sleep). During stage 2 sleep, short episodes of increased activity, called "sleep spindles," are observed on the electroencephalogram. Gradually stage 2 sleep disappears and even slower waves and higher voltage are observed on the EEG, signifying stage 3 sleep. Finally, the elder enters the deepest stage of sleep, stage 4. During stage 4 sleep, one can observe large slow waves of high voltage at a frequency of 1½ to 2 cycles per second. Breathing and heart rate are also slow and the elder can be awakened only with difficulty.

After reaching the deepest stage of sleep, the sleeping elder retraces the stages, progressing from stage 4 to stage 3, to stage 2 and then, approximately 1½ hours into the night, the sleeper enters the first episode of dream or rapid eye movement (REM) sleep, which coincides with stage 1. This period of sleep is unique, in that breathing becomes more rapid, heart rate increases, blood pressure is elevated, and body temperature changes. These responses are probably a physical correlate of the process of dreaming. When electrodes are placed near the muscles that move the eyes, the eye movements recorded are similar to those in individuals who are awake, moving rapidly from one side to the other. During non-REM sleep (stages 2 to 4) the eyes move slowly and in a circular pattern. The paradox of rapid eye movement or dream sleep is that the voluntary muscles are almost completely paralyzed despite the increased activity of the brain. Only the most extreme effort can move the arms or legs during REM sleep. Possibly, there is a blockage at the base of the brain that prohibits transmission of electrical impulses to the muscles and subsequently protects us from injury during the stage of sleep when the brain is producing the unusual and occasionally frightening images of dreams.

Other phenomena occur during the process of dream or REM sleep. The internal control of body temperature decreases and therefore body temperature tends to rise or fall in parallel with the surrounding environment (Marsh et al., 1987). Our capacity to hear permits us to respond to loud sounds during REM sleep. Even the sexual organs respond during REM sleep. For example, males often experience penile erections during dream sleep. These erections are not usually associated with an explicit sexual dream. That males experience erections during REM sleep permits a unique diagnostic test. Some older men fear that they have lost their ability to develop and maintain an erection because of physical changes. By attaching a strain gauge to the penis during the night and tracing the size and rigidity of the penis in conjunction with the stages of sleep, it can be determined if the lack of ability during wakeful hours to obtain and maintain an erection continues during sleep. Frequently, the older man who fears impotence does experience erections during the night, suggesting that psychological treatment for sexual impotence is appropriate.

As suggested above, the stages of sleep are influenced by underlying rhythms that control, to a considerable extent, all biologic activities. This rhythm is the rest-activity cycle (Marsh et al., 1987). The basic rest and activity cycle generally lasts about ninety minutes and repeats itself throughout the day and night. During this cycle, elders fluctuate from wakefulness to lethargy. The cycle occurs as the elder progresses through all of the stages of sleep, and it begins anew about every ninety minutes. Therefore, the elder will experience approximately five of these cycles per night.

Another basic rhythm is the circadian rhythm. This twenty-four-hour rhythm controls many biologic functions. One of these functions is the period during the day when a person feels lethargic and tired, versus those periods when he or she is wakeful and energetic. In addition, circadian cycles control those periods of deepest sleep. For example, for most people the early hours of sleep are when the deepest sleep occurs and are characterized by less frequent and prolonged episodes of REM, or dream, sleep. In contrast, as the morning approaches, REM sleep intensifies and one is more likely to be awakened by dreams (frequently awakening for the last time from a dream). Body temperature tends to reach its highest level just past the middle of the awakening period and reaches its lowest level in the middle of the sleeping period. As noted above, changing environments and changing the time of sleep disrupt the circadian rhythms. Factors that tend to control and reset circadian rhythms include exposure to bright sunlight, exercise, and diet.

CHANGES IN THE SLEEP CYCLE WITH AGING

A number of changes occur with aging in the normal sleep patterns. For one, the relative amount of dream sleep decreases as individuals age, from over 40 percent in early childhood to about 25 percent by the age of 70. Some disease states are characterized by even more prominent decreases in REM sleep, such as Alzheimer's disease. Slow wave (stage 4) sleep decreases with age as well. Some elders experience no episodes of slow wave sleep during a night (or only one episode very early in the sleep cycle). The significance of the loss of slow wave sleep is not known. Older persons require more time to fall asleep once the lights have turned out (though this is not dramatic, ranging from three to five minutes for younger adults to eight to ten minutes for older adults).

Arousals, though they occur at all ages, are more frequent in the elderly than in middle-aged adults. Most persons do not recognize the number of times they are aroused during the night, for the person must remain awake for at least a minute or two in order to remember that he or she awakened. As older persons tend to be aroused for longer periods of time, they remember more awakenings. Yet the time lost from sleep by these awakenings is relatively small (though very disturbing to the elder). For example, an older person may awaken four or five times during the night for no longer than three to five minutes on each occasion (a total of fifteen to twenty minutes). Nevertheless, the elder perceives that sleep has been seriously hampered and that hours have been spent awake during the night. If an older person must leave the bed to urinate on one or two occasions during the night, he or she will be more aroused and will usually remember the number of times that he or she awakens, reinforcing a sense of poor sleep. The process of returning to sleep takes longer after being aroused by walking to the bathroom.

In general, older sleepers will report that their sleep has been less refreshing and that they experience more lethargy in the morning than younger adults. Because of their concern regarding sleep, older adults spend more time in bed when they are not asleep, hoping to catch a few extra moments of sleep. Investigators of sleep have coined the term "sleep efficiency," that is, the time actually spent asleep divided by the time spent in bed. Whereas young persons achieve a sleep efficiency of 90 to 95 percent, the sleep efficiency of the elder is on average around 70 percent. Snoring tends to increase in frequency with age. Among persons over the age of 75 in one study, over 50 percent reported snoring (compared to less than 10 percent for adolescents).

THE BIOLOGIC CAUSES OF INSOMNIA IN LATE LIFE

What are the causes of insomnia and the other sleep difficulties in older persons? Some investigators suggest that the structural brain changes that accompany the aging process, those same changes that affect memory and intelligence, also affect sleep. The evidence supporting the suggestion derives from studies of the sleep of persons suffering dementia (in some ways an exaggeration of the normal brain changes that occur with aging, though dementia certainly is not an extension of the aging process). Persons suffering dementia take longer to fall asleep, suffer more awakenings during the night, and experience less stage 4 sleep.

A second cause of sleep problems among the elderly is disruption of the circadian rhythms or the biological clock. These biological clocks appear to become disrupted in late life. Sleep may be redistributed across the twenty-four-hour day, with elders retiring earlier in the evening, awakening earlier in the morning and sleeping more frequently during the day. Some elders even resemble infants who enter multiple episodes of sleep during the day. Older persons are probably less tolerant of the inevitable phase shifts that are required in the sleep-wake cycle when one must stay awake for a period of time, travel across time zones, or is awakened for some reason during the evening. If the elder is forced to remain in bed for an extended time due to an illness or injury (such as a fractured hip), the supine position further disrupts sleep.

THE PSYCHOLOGICAL CAUSES OF INSOMNIA
IN LATE LIFE

Psychological factors can also disrupt the sleep cycle. Persons suffering anxiety will often have difficulty falling asleep initially, but once asleep, usually are capable of sleeping through the night. The depressed, as described in Chapter 4, suffer frequent nightly and early morning awakenings, although they rarely have difficulty in falling asleep. The disruption of sleep with depression and dementia simulates the normal changes of sleep with aging. Through careful analysis of the electroencephalogram and other sleep monitors, a distinction can be made, however. Worry about sleep or anticipation of stressful or even pleasurable events the next day also disrupts sleep.

Social and cultural factors also contribute to sleep problems suffered by the elderly. A "good night's sleep" is greatly valued in our society. Most believe eight hours of sleep is necessary for proper functioning. Many plan activities based upon the unrealistic expectation that persons of all ages require eight hours of sleep and will not awaken during the night. Therefore, attendants in long-term care facilities often discourage older persons from arising during the evening and encourage them to remain in bed for eight hours. The older adult subsequently believes that his or her sleep is abnormal, despite the fact that the actual sleep pattern and time spent asleep may be normal, given the age of the individual. This concern, in turn, leads to the excessive use of medications, especially the sedative/hypnotic agents. Sedatives are often prescribed because the nature of sleep in the elderly is poorly understood by clinicians, family members, and caregivers. These drugs may actually contribute to further disruption of the biologic patterns of sleep and therefore complicate sleep difficulties to an even greater extent than prior to the prescription of the medication. They may also lead to a psychological dependence on the drugs and a fear that the elder cannot sleep without medication.

The Diagnostic Workup

Clinicians biologically evaluate sleep disorders using the polysomnographic, or sleep, study. These studies can be performed at specialized centers throughout the country, which are usually called "sleep disorder centers." Polysomnography means "multiple monitoring of sleep." The basic recording of the polysomnogram is the electroencephalogram (EEG), which is a record of background electrical activity from the brain. As described earlier, electrical activity changes during sleep, and these changes allow clinicians to label the stages of sleep.

A second recording of the polysomnogram is an electromyogram—an electrode placed near the eyes of an individual to record movement of the eyes (recording the electrical activity of muscles that move the eyes). From the measure of eye movement, REM sleep can be distinguished from non-REM sleep. A third component of the polysomnogram records both movement of the chest (in respirations per minute) and air flow. The measure of air flow enables the clinician to determine if oxygen is passing regularly into the lungs and subsequently to the brain and other parts of the body. Chest movements help determine whether the breathing mechanism continues throughout the night. The evaluation of breathing is essential to the diagnosis of the sleep apneas. In an obstructive sleep apnea, respirations actually increase but air flow decreases (because of the blockage in the upper airway). In central sleep apnea, air flow decreases as do respirations.

Other investigators place electrodes on the extremities of the individual during sleep to record periodic movements of the legs. Still others record blood pressure. These multiple measures viewed simultaneously enable the sleep specialist to diagnose and differentiate the sleep disorders described. One or two hours are required for the sleep tracings to be reviewed by the clinician. Investigators are beginning to use computers to evaluate these tracings (especially to evaluate the progression from one stage of sleep to another on the electroencephalogram).

The psychological evaluation of sleep disorders requires a thorough in-person interview of not only the older adult suffering a sleep problem but a family member, preferably a sleep partner. The elder should be questioned regarding the hours of sleep each night, the time required from turning out the lights to falling asleep, the number of awakenings during the night, the number of times the elder goes to the bathroom, the usual time of final awakening in the morning, and the amount of time spent in bed following awakening in the morning. To assist the older person in providing this information to the clinician, a sleep-wake diary can be kept for one to two weeks. Given the concern of older persons about their sleep difficulties, they often exaggerate or misinterpret the amount of time asleep versus the amount of time awake. In addition, the number of naps taken during the day should be noted.

In addition to a thorough characterization of the sleep-wake cycle, the elder should be questioned regarding medications, diet, exercise during the day, experiences of lethargy, periods during the day when he or she feels most active, and periods of the day when he or she feels drowsy. Sudden versus gradual changes in the sleep pattern should be determined. Many persons have experienced difficulties with their sleep for most of their adult life and the problems presented by the older person suffering sleep difficulties are not new but become of concern only in late life.

Following the interview of the family, a decision must be made as to whether a sleep study is to be performed. These studies are expensive and inconvenient (although they are more convenient now than a few years ago). In more advanced sleep laboratories, patients are fitted with portable monitors and are allowed to return home (or possibly to a hotel room) for the sleep tracing. At least two nights of sleep monitoring are required for an accurate sleep study. All medication should be stopped that might affect sleep (such as antidepressant medication, tranquilizers, and especially sleeping pills) for at least seven to ten days beforehand. The inconvenience and the cost of sleep studies necessitate the careful screening of elders in order to determine who actually needs to undergo a study.

Patients who are known to snore by report of a family member and who have difficulty staying awake during the day are prime candidates for a sleep study. Headaches in the morning, a restless sleep, and memory impairment reinforce the need of such a study. The sleep investigator will be attempting to determine if sleep apnea is present. Any patient over the age of 40 who complains of sleep problems for over three months could benefit from a sleep study, especially those individuals who have attempted to correct the problem with good sleep hygiene, yet the insomnia persists. Patients with the restless leg syndrome or periodic leg movements also are candidates for a sleep study.

Treatment for Sleep Disorders

Clinicians should always be attentive to underlying causes of sleep problems, for these problems often mask others. As mentioned frequently throughout this book, anxiety, fear, grief, depression, or confusion all contribute to sleep difficulties.

SLEEP HYGIENE

To correct sleep disorders in older adults, the clinician should begin by recommending a program of good sleep hygiene to the elder. Medications should only be used after attempts to improve the milieu of sleep have failed or when the sleep difficulty can be attributed to a specific psychiatric or physical problem (such as major depression). As a rule, persons should be encouraged to sleep as much as required in order to be refreshed the following day, but no more. The amount of sleep necessary varies from one person to another despite the tendency for less sleep to be required with increasing age. If elders cannot fall asleep, they should be encouraged to get out of bed until they feel drowsy enough to return to bed. Excessive time in bed reinforces a shallow restless sleep with frequent awakenings.

For persons suffering sleep difficulties, a regular schedule of sleep is essential. The time for awakening is more important to regulate than the time one turns off the lights. Each morning, the person should get out of bed at approximately the same time, whether it is during the week or on the weekend. For older persons not constricted by schedules, encouraging such regimentation (which reminds the elder of years of work when he or she had to adhere to schedules) can be distasteful. Nevertheless, a regular time of awakening in the morning will eventually regulate the time of sleep onset.

If the older person is physically healthy, daily exercise can improve sleep. Exercise should be regular and not pursued during the evening. Exercising prior to bedtime activates the body (as well as the mind) and even though the elder may feel tired, he or she may find it difficult to fall asleep after exercising. Excessive exercise of the legs and arms can lead to restlessness or aches and pain that can interrupt sleep. Therefore, a moderate exercise program focused on cardiopulmonary function is recommended instead of body-building. Walking, cycling, and swimming are excellent exercises for older adults.

The bedroom of the sleep-deprived older adult should be adjusted to maximize sleep. First, extraneous, intermittent noise should be reduced (by using carpets, curtains, and even soundproof doors). Economics may not always permit the older person to insulate a room against noise, especially when the elder lives in a busy city or perhaps cannot afford air conditioning and therefore must leave windows open during the summer. The use of "white noise"—steady background noise—can help in such a situation. For example, a person may keep a fan running, even during the winter, though the fan should not be pointed toward the bed. During the winter, a "white noise" generator can be purchased for around $100 and uses less electricity than a fan. The room should be kept as dark as possible, though a night light may be necessary to ensure safety when the elder must arise to go to the bathroom. As noted earlier, a digital clock should be pointed away from the person so that he or she cannot remember the times at which awakening occurs during the night.

A moderately cool room temperature promotes better sleep. Sixty-eight to seventy degrees is optimal during the summer and the room can be cooled even more during the winter (when sufficient bed covering is available). The room should be cooled for an hour prior to going to bed so that significant changes do not occur in temperature once the elder begins sleep.

A number of behaviors prior to bedtime can facilitate improved sleep in elders suffering sleep problems. Excessive liquids should be avoided in the evening to decrease the need for trips to the bathroom during the night. Caffeinated beverages are to be avoided in the evening, as are analgesic medications that contain caffeine. If the elder enjoys a nighttime cup of coffee or tea, the use of a decaffeinated coffee or tea or an herbal tea can be substituted for regular coffee or tea. A light snack at bedtime assists in decreasing hunger, which may disturb sleep. A heavy meal, however, can lead to discomfort during the night. Alcohol is not a useful sedative in the sleep-disordered elder. Because of the short life of alcohol in the body, the initial sedative effects wear off in three to four hours and the elder experiences a rebound arousal during the middle of the night.

As previously described, persons who cannot fall asleep should not remain in bed and "fight sleep." Some elders are so determined to fall asleep that they become angry and frustrated as they try harder and harder to fall asleep, thus paradoxically increasing arousal. Rather, the older person should leave the bedroom and concentrate on a completely different task to take one's mind away from the sleep problem. A nonstimulating, boring book encourages drowsiness. When drowsiness ensues, the elder can then return to the bedroom. Regardless of how little sleep is forthcoming during the night, the older person should continue to arise at the same time each morning.

Chronic tobacco use also contributes to sleep difficulties. Therefore, if the older person is suffering sleep problems, arising and going to another room for a cigarette may further complicate the problem. If an elder is undergoing a withdrawal from tobacco (because of health or other reason), sleep may be disturbed temporarily but eventually will become better than when the elder was smoking.

Therapists working with elders suffering insomnia can assist sleep by recommending appropriate sleep hygiene as described above. In addition, clinicians should take a supportive stance. Although sleep problems may not be considered by a busy physician to be worthy of the attention that more serious health problems require, nevertheless they can be very disturbing to an older adult. Time spent with the elder empathizing with the frustration and lethargy that result from sleep difficulties and explaining the normal variances of sleep is time well spent. The clinician may also teach relaxation techniques when tension and restlessness are problems during the onset of sleep. If, however, the older person has no difficulty with falling asleep but frequent awakenings are the problem, relaxation techniques are of little value.

PHARMACOLOGIC THERAPY

The biologic treatment of sleep dates back many centuries. Drugs such as laudanum, alcohol, and various herbs have been reported to produce stupor or relaxation. Yet most were too unpredictable to be universally accepted to promote the much-desired sleep. Bromides were among the first hypnotics to be regularly prescribed. Of the other drugs prescribed before the twentieth century, only chloryl hydrate and paraldehyde are still used today. Phenobarbitol, introduced during the first decade of the twentieth century, was the first drug to be prescribed consistently for sleep. Since that time, many agents have been recommended for inducing and maintaining sleep (Harvey, 1980).

The use of barbiturates such as phenobarbital for sleep induction and maintenance is rarely indicated today (Reynolds et al., 1985). Secobarbital (Seconal) and pentobarbital (Nembutal) were the barbiturates prescribed most often, but are no longer the drugs of choice for sleep. The barbiturates cause physical and psychological dependence and are potentially lethal if the number of pills in a usual prescription bottle are taken all at once. This dosage suppresses respiration enough to kill a person during a suicide attempt. Only chloral hydrate, a short-acting barbiturate, is still used regularly at present. This drug is relatively safe and can be used for short periods of time, especially within the hospital. The drug provides a useful sedative effect when given in a dose of 500 mg once or twice at night, for it rarely interferes with other medications or biologic tests that are performed in the hospital. Given its potential for lethality and physical dependence, however, chloral hydrate should not be prescribed outside the hospital.

The medications most often used for sleep today fall into the benzodiazepine category. Three of these agents are well known: flurazepam (Dalmane), temazepam (Restoril), and triazolam (Halcion). Flurazepam is the longest-acting of the agents, usually given in a dose of 15 to 30 mg at night. In older adults, the drug may work well for a short period of time as a sedative but eventually leads to increased difficulties with sleep. In addition, the older adult may experience significant problems the next day with confusion. Therefore, most physicians prescribe shorter-acting agents. Temazepam is a shorter-acting agent, the dosage being the same as that for flurazepam. The shortest-acting of the current agents available is triazolam; it is given in a dose between 0.125 and 0.25 mg. If triazolam is given in a higher dose, significant side effects such as confusion, amnesia, impaired coordination, and slurred speech may occur.

The benzodiazepines are useful for treating insomnia, especially insomnia secondary to anxiety. There is a significant potential, however, for physical dependence and even more for psychological dependence. Many people believe they require the medication for sleep when in fact they do not. In contrast to the barbiturates, there is much less potential for a lethal overdose (though successful suicides have been completed with the amount of pills usually prescribed) and the benzodiazepines have relatively few side effects.

Many other drugs are available for treating sleep and some will be reviewed briefly. Diphenhydramine hydrochloride (Benadryl) is an anticholinergic and antihistaminic agent. Antihistamines (cold medications) make one drowsy and therefore can induce sleep. Nevertheless, Benadryl is not a true sedative and will not correct the more severe sleep disorders. L-Tryptophan, an amino acid, can be bought over-the-counter (although it is somewhat expensive) and is used frequently as a sedative. The drug has virtually no side effects but also has much less potential for inducing and maintaining sleep than a traditional sedative hypnotic agent. Aspirin also may be a useful sedative agent if it is not combined with caffeine. Aspirin appears to increase the concentration of serotonin in the brain and increased concentrations of serotonin have been associated with improved sleep.

Principles for prescribing sedative agents are as follows:

1. First, an adequate attempt to improve sleep hygiene is indicated before such medications are prescribed.
2. Sedatives should be used only for a short period of time (two to three weeks and then discontinued).
3. The lowest possible effective dose should be prescribed (often one-third to one-half that prescribed for younger patients).
4. Patients should take the medications approximately thirty minutes prior to bedtime and bedtime should be the same every night.
5. Patients should be encouraged to maintain good sleep hygiene in addition to the use of medications.
6. Even if chronic use appears indicated, patients should not take the medication every night. Rather, they may be given ten to twenty pills per month and be instructed to distribute the medication over the month (such as using the medication every other night). Most persons can

tolerate some insomnia if they know that at least every other night they can sleep relatively well.

References

American Psychological Association. *Diagnostic and Statistical Manual of Mental Disorders* (3d ed.). Washington, DC: American Psychological Association, 1987.

Dement, W. C., L. E. Miles, and M. A. Carskadon. "White paper on sleeping and aging." *Journal of the American Geriatric Society*, 30:25, 1982.

Freud, S. *Introductory Lectures on Psychoanalysis*. London: Hogarth Press, 1917.

Harvey, S. C. "Hypnotics and sedatives." In A. G. Gilman, L. S. Goodman, and A. Gilman (Eds.), *Goodman and Gilman's The Pharmacological Basis of Therapeutics*. New York: Macmillan, 1980. Pp. 339–375.

Lugaresi, E., M. Zucconi, and E. O. Bixler. "Epidemiology of sleep disorders." *Psychiatric Annals*, 17:446, 1987.

Marsh, G. R., T. J. Hoelscher, C. W. Erwin, and M. D. Web. "Sleep: Its nature and alteration with age." *Center Reports on Advances in Research*, 11:1, 1987.

Mosko, S. S., M. J. Dickel, P. Paul, et al. "Sleep apnea and sleep-related periodic leg movements in community resident seniors." *Journal of the American Geriatric Society*, 36:502, 1988.

Reynolds, C. F., D. J. Kupfer, C. C. Hoch, and D. E. Sewitch. "Sleeping pills for the elderly: Are they ever justified?" *Journal of Clinical Psychiatry*, 46:9, 1985.

Suggested Reading

Borberly, A. *Secrets of Sleep*. New York: Basic Books, 1986.

Hartmann, N. E. *The Sleep Book: Understanding and Preventing Sleep Problems in People Over 50*. Glenview, IL: Scott, Foresman, and Co., 1987.

CHAPTER NINE

Alcohol and Drug Abuse

The use of alcohol is as old as Western civilization. Persons in ancient times looked upon alcohol as "the water of life" and provided it with magical significance in not only social but also religious ceremonies. Even today, we toast "the health" of others with alcohol (Maddox and Blazer, 1985). Dionysus, the mythological son of the Greek god Zeus, was the god of the vine and wine. He was born of fire and nursed by rain (the heat that ripens the grapes and the water that keeps the plant alive). The god of wine could be kind and beneficent or cruel and drive people to terrible deeds, such as causing the Theban women to attack Pentheus and tear him limb from limb.

The dual nature of Dionysus reflects even today the conflicting views regarding the use of alcohol in Western society. Though alcohol remains the recreational beverage of choice for good times and social "mixers," the drug is potentially toxic and addictive. Acute alcohol intoxication has been implicated in as many as 50 percent of all traffic fatalities. As many as 5 percent of all adult drinkers are thought to be alcohol dependent and thus represent a major public health problem.

In many ways, the use and abuse of other psychoactive drugs by elders, especially the abuse of tranquilizers and sedative/hypnotic agents, mirror the use and abuse of alcohol, although the acceptance of these drugs among persons who would never consider drinking alcohol is an interesting paradox. Most tranquilizing and sedative drugs used by older adults are not perceived as "recreational" and admitted drug abuse is uncommon among the elderly. Even so, 25 percent of the medications (both prescription and over-the-counter) used in this country are consumed by persons 65 years of age and older, which is 2.5 times more than would be expected given the percentage of the population. Though many of these agents are for the treatment of chronic medical illnesses (such as high blood pressure or osteoarthritis), sleeping pills and tranquilizers are among the more frequent drugs used by older adults.

The prevalence of alcohol abuse and/or dependence ranges from about 2 to 5 percent for men and is less than 1 percent for women over the age of 65 (Blazer and Pennybacker, 1984). Both the current frequency of alcohol problems in late life and the lifetime frequency of problems among the current cohort of elders are lower than for younger persons. This difference is explained in part by lifetime differences in drinking patterns in the current generation of elders compared to current younger adults. In addition, survivors into late life may overrepresent individuals who have remained abstinent from alcohol through much of their life or have only been moderate drinkers. Total abstinence from alcohol is more frequent among the elderly than for any other age group. In a survey by Armor et al. (1977), 52 percent of elderly men and 68 percent of elderly women were current abstainers. These percentages will drop as younger birth cohorts who have more frequently used alcohol enter late life during the latter twentieth and early twenty-first century.

Despite the lower relative use of alcohol among older adults and the infrequent use of recreational drugs (such as cocaine), drug abuse problems do arise among elders related to abuse and dependence on alcohol and prescribed drugs. Stresses on older adults may, on occasion, precipitate either the beginning of alcohol/drug use or an increase in alcohol/drug use among persons previously free of problems from alcohol and drugs. A decreased ability to process (metabolize) alcohol and eliminate the drug from the body coupled with the toxic effects of alcohol on a number of organs precipitate both medical and emotional problems with alcohol in individuals who do not change their pattern of alcohol intake through time. When spouses and children do not expect their elderly family members to develop problems from alcohol or drug use, the recognition of abuse is blunted. The following case examples illustrate the types of problems that professionals face with alcohol and drug abuse. Most of the principles for diagnosis and intervention apply equally to prescription drug abuse.

Mr. Phillipson was a nationally recognized construction engineer. As a designer of bridges and consultant to many groups throughout the country regarding the relative strength of various bridge designs, he enjoyed a comfortable yet active professional and social life. Yet Mr. Phillipson was not a unidimensional man. For years, he had an abiding interest in the theater (though he did not act). Given his knowledge of the theater, the local newspaper asked him to regularly review local productions. His reviews of plays appeared about once per month in the newspaper and he thoroughly enjoyed writing the review column.

Given his eclectic interests and affable personality, Mr. Phillipson attended local country clubs and other social gatherings two to three times a week most of his adult years. From early adulthood, he drank "socially" at these gatherings. His regular alcohol consumption included a cocktail or two upon returning home from his work, a glass of wine for dinner, and a drink or two the nights that he and his wife attended the various social gatherings to which they were invited.

Mr. Phillipson's wife was concerned that her husband was suffering some problems with his memory. Phillipson himself admitted that memory became a problem during his mid-sixties and therefore he retired from consulting work, for he feared that his decrease in logic and reasoning might endanger the construction of a bridge. Nevertheless, he continued to frequent the theater and write his monthly reviews. He often attended meetings with fellow engineers and had no difficulty in maintaining a conversation with them. At home, however, he became anxious, for he no longer could recall quickly the location of his stocks and bonds and the amount in his current bank account. Phillipson had always suffered anxiety about money, fearing that he would become impoverished, even though he admitted that he and his wife had more than an adequate income.

Upon consultation with his local physician, Mr. Phillipson was referred to a psychiatrist for an evaluation of his memory difficulties.

Upon arrival at the psychiatrist's office, he was well dressed and groomed and most pleasant in his conversation. Upon routine memory assessment, Mr. Phillipson exhibited no major difficulties but did fail two minor tests (recent recall and proverb abstraction). This failure disturbed him. He was referred for psychological testing. Test results suggested that Phillipson suffered a significant memory loss that was typical of cognitive problems from chronic alcohol use. Neurologic examination was normal.

Mr. Phillipson had great difficulty in accepting that alcohol was the cause of his problem. Alcohol had meant much to him through his life. The cocktail that he drank before supper was a highlight of the day—a symbol that he could relax and prepare himself for an enjoyable evening with his friends and colleagues. When the test results were explained to him and his wife, she affirmed the severity of the alcohol problem and revealed that she had, for years, feared that Mr. Phillipson was drinking more than he should.

For six months the psychiatrist suggested plans to withdraw Mr. Phillipson from alcohol. He refused to admit the association of alcohol use and memory problems, for his memory problem was not that severe and he did not appreciate being controlled in his behavior. Then he suffered an automobile accident and while admitted to the hospital (unknown to the psychiatrist at the time), he became acutely delirious. Only after 48 hours of agitation and hallucinations was it discovered by the attending physician that Mr. Phillipson was suffering from acute alcohol withdrawal with delirium tremens. He was treated with a tranquilizer, diazepam, and withdrawn from alcohol while in the hospital. This event convinced Mr. Phillipson and he stopped drinking. His memory problems improved somewhat (though not enough that he could return to his former occupation). He continued to regret losing the social pleasure of a cocktail which had been greatly valued through most of his adult life.

 Mrs. Carteret was an elderly married woman from the coastal region of North Carolina. She had lived a life similar to many of her upper middle-class companions, attended church regularly, and had been abstinent from alcohol all of her life. She began to experience some problems with her nerves when she was 60 years old and was prescribed a little white pill (meprobamate [Miltown]). If she took this medicine in the morning, she felt much better during the day. Therefore she took the drug and thought little of it. A few years later she began to suffer sleeping problems. Her physician, after suggesting that her sleep problem was not serious, prescribed flurazepam (Dalmane) 15 mg at night. She slept well for a while but her sleep gradually deteriorated and she required a larger dose (30 mg) and often would repeat the 30 mg dose at least once during the night.

Because of increased concern with her sleep, Mrs. Carteret became more nervous during the day, worried that she would not sleep at night. The little white pill, as it worked so well in the morning, was taken two, three, or four times a day. She was embarrassed that she was forced to take medication so often and, to avoid what she perceived to be a lecture from her physician, was able to obtain a second prescription from a specialist treating her for arthritic pains at a medical center some miles away. Still a third physician, an ophthalmologist, whom she had consulted about possible cataracts, prescribed flurazepam for sleep as well, unaware that her family physician was also prescribing the drug.

When she was 72, Mrs. Carteret's family began to notice that she was lethargic and even appeared intoxicated on occasions. They searched the house for alcohol (as her father had been an alcoholic) but found no evidence of alcohol. Mrs. Carteret vehemently denied that she would ever touch alcohol because of the terrible example set by her father. Upon searching the house, however, the family discovered many pill bottles for meprobamate and flurazepam. They referred her to a local physician who attempted to withdraw her from the drugs as an outpatient over two weeks under the control of the family. Mrs. Carteret's anxiety became so severe, however, that she could not tolerate the withdrawal, thus forcing hospitalization.

During a ten-day hospitalization, Mrs. Carteret was successfully withdrawn from meprobamate and flurazepam. At the end of the ten days, however, she was experiencing considerable problems with her sleep and was extremely anxious. She begged the physicians to help her and did not believe herself strong enough to tolerate the lack of the medications. She remained in the hospital an additional ten days and gradually the anxiety subsided without the aid of medications. The family was warned of the seriousness of the use of these drugs by Mrs. Carteret and even the patient appeared convinced when she was discharged from the hospital that the medication had become a major problem. Her anxiety persisted, but six months following hospitalization she had not returned to either the sleeping pills or the little white pill.

Alcohol-Related Problems

Alcoholism most often produces a clinical picture of abuse, dependence, or both. In recent studies, the distinction between the two groups, especially when they are observed through time, are virtually nil (Blazer and Siegler, 1984). Older adults suffering alcohol dependence may take more drinks per day and suffer more medical problems, yet abuse and dependence are so often interrelated that they can be considered the same disorder.

The three classic patterns of alcohol abuse are: regular daily intake of large amounts of alcohol (sometimes two pints a day); regular heavy drinking limited to weekends or social events; and long periods of abstinence from alcohol intermixed with binges of heavy drinking every day lasting for days or weeks (Goodwin and Guzes, 1989).

To determine if a person is suffering alcohol dependence, the CAGE questions (Bernadt et al., 1982) are useful for screening, but they are not as applicable in late life as in other stages of the life cycle. These questions include:

C—Have you felt the need to Cut down on your drinking?
A—Have you ever felt Annoyed by criticism of your drinking?
G—Have you had Guilty feelings about drinking?
E—Have you ever taken a morning Eyeopener?

Older persons are more likely to expose their alcohol problems to the family or clinician by physical and psychological symptoms of persistent drinking as opposed to personal guilt or concern about drinking. Many older persons may not even recognize the connection between emerging physical or emotional problems (such as difficulty sleeping) and their drinking habits which have continued for many decades.

Other alcohol-related problems in late life besides abuse and dependence do occur. The most common is *alcohol intoxication*. The symptoms of intoxication—slurred speech, uncoordination, an unsteady gait, a flushed face, poor judgment, and a labile mood—are easy to distinguish regardless of age. The evidence of the intoxicating agent is easily identified and, if the older adult is not chronically addicted to alcohol, withdrawal leads to full recovery (but not without discomfort). The degree of intoxication can be monitored by obtaining alcohol levels in the blood. Some older adults appear intoxicated with blood levels as low as 30 mg/dl, though most become intoxicated at blood levels over 75 mg/dl. If the blood level exceeds 400 mg/di, the person's life may be threatened. Acute intoxication is often associated with (and revealed by) alcohol-related problems, such as an automobile accident, a violent outburst, a fall or accident, excessive exposure to heat or cold, or self-destructive behavior.

Alcohol withdrawal usually leads to tremors, weakness, sweating, an elevated blood pressure, an elevated heart rate, a depressed mood, headache, dry mouth, and difficulty sleeping. The symptoms generally cease after 12 to 24 hours. A more severe form of alcohol withdrawal may develop—*delirium tremens*. The symptoms of alcohol withdrawal become more severe in alcohol withdrawal delirium; the onset is usually two to three days after cessation or a reduction in alcohol intake (as opposed to a few hours after the last drink in the usual alcohol withdrawal syndrome). If not treated effectively, the delusions, agitated behavior, fever, and seizures that accompany alcohol withdrawal delirium can be life threatening.

Some older adults develop an *alcoholic hallucinosis*. In this condition, vivid and persistent visual hallucinations develop usually within 24 hours after stopping or reducing alcohol intake. The auditory hallucinations are usually voices and are experienced as unpleasant, if not frightening. Unlike delirium tremens, alcoholic hallucinosis may persist for many days or even weeks after alcohol withdrawal.

A severe problem associated with alcohol ingestion is memory loss. The *alcoholic amnestics disorder* is characterized by difficulty with both short- and long-term memory and an inability to learn new information. The elder may not be able to tell the clinician what happened the day before, what he ate for breakfast, where he was born, or well-known facts, such as past presidents or special dates. The amnestic syndrome usually develops after prolonged and heavy intake of alcohol and is due to a deficiency in thiamine (vitamin B_1). The alcoholic amnestic disorder is also known as Korsakoff's syndrome. The disorder may follow an acute period of confusion and other symptoms of nervous system dysfunction, including a loss of balance (ataxia). This acute episode, often called *Wernicke's encephalopathy*, usually subsides, but if the disorder is not treated with supplemental thiamine, the alcoholic amnestic disorder will emerge. A long-term dementia associated with alcoholism (with symptoms similar to the dementias described in Chapter 2) may also develop in individuals who maintain chronic alcohol use over many years.

Abuse of and addiction to other substances by older adults usually consists of drugs prescribed by physicians or psychoactive agents that can be bought at a pharmacy or grocery store. These substances range from caffeine (as a stimulant) to the sedative/ hypnotic and tranquilizing drugs. Among older adults, abuse of tranquilizing and sedative/hypnotic agents is the most common abuse observed. The psychoactive substances are taken in larger amounts over longer periods of time (though an older adult may begin to experience the symptoms of abuse by taking the same amount with the body gradually less capable of metabolizing the drug). The elder may recognize the need to attempt to control use of the drug, especially a sleeping pill, but may be unable to reduce or control use of the drug. He or she may "doctor shop" to maintain a supply of the medication or borrow medications from family and friends. Withdrawal symptoms from the tranquilizers and sedative/ hypnotics are similar to those of withdrawal from alcohol. Excessive use or abuse of the sedative/hypnotics and tranquilizers produce symptoms similar to alcohol intoxication.

The Etiology of Alcohol and Drug Use Problems in Late Life

A number of biologic theories have been developed to explain the severe disability that results from alcohol consumption among a small segment of the population whereas a majority of the population can use the beverage without difficulty (Blazer, 1989). Genetic or hereditary factors have received the most attention in these studies. Children of alcoholics, in a series of studies performed in Scandinavian countries, were found to be four times more likely than children of nonalcoholics to suffer alcoholism as adults. This increased frequency of alcohol problems in children persisted even when the children were not raised by their natural parents.

The Scandinavian countries provide a unique opportunity to study this phenomenon, for during the impoverished years of the first part of this century, many children were separated from their natural parents and were adopted. In a Swedish study, nearly one-fourth of adopted male alcoholics had biologic fathers who suffered alcoholism. Identical (or monozygotic) twins were nearly twice as likely to suffer concordant alcoholism than fraternal (or dizygotic) twins. Unfortunately, few of these studies have considered alcoholism that appears for the first time in late life. Alcoholics who survive into late life after years of abuse and dependence clearly exhibit this genetic predisposition to the development of alcohol problems.

Other biologic theories of alcohol relate more to the interaction between the aging process and the absorption, distribution, and metabolism of alcohol by the older adult. If the elder maintains a constant intake of alcohol through the retirement years and the complete absorption of alcohol persists, the potential for increased toxic effects may appear for the first time in late life, thus creating a vicious cycle of increasingly toxic levels of alcohol and a decreasing capacity to physically manage the alcohol. Most investigators find that alcohol absorption (rapid earlier in life) continues to be rapid and complete into late life. Though food in the stomach, such as milk products, retards absorption, many alcoholics drink instead of eating and therefore quickly become intoxicated by even small amounts of alcohol.

Alcohol is distributed throughout the body of the older adult. Elders have less total body water, less extracellular fluid, and a higher percentage of body fat. As alcohol does not distribute to fatty tissue, the net effect is that the same dose of alcohol ingested by an older person compared to a younger person of the same weight leads to a higher fluid concentration in the older adult.

Alcohol in the body is almost totally oxidized (one of the first steps in metabolism) by the liver. The enzyme alcohol dehydrogenase performs this task and this enzyme decreases in effectiveness as persons increase in age. Throughout the life cycle, the metabolism of alcohol is slow and predictable. For this reason, maintenance of a given blood level of alcohol through steady intake over time is essential, otherwise intoxication or withdrawal symptoms appear. Long-term alcoholics recognize this characteristic of alcohol use and therefore "pace" their drinking. The rate of intake must be slowed as individuals age to avoid the effects, yet most elderly alcoholics do not recognize this change.

Many psychological problems also contribute to the increased use of alcohol in late life. Alcohol is a readily available and moderately effective means of decreasing anxiety. As problems with anxiety may emerge for the first time in the elderly, alcohol use can increase in older adults suffering from anxiety symptoms. Persons who are withdrawn, isolated, impulsive, and hypersensitive are especially at risk for the use of alcohol. The so-called addictive personality leads to just as great a risk for alcohol and drug use in late life as at other stages of the life cycle.

Stressful events also contribute to the onset of alcohol problems. Concurrent psychiatric disorders contribute as well. In a recent study, 81 percent of the persons who experienced the onset of alcoholism later in life experienced a stressor associated with the alcohol use (Finlayson et al., 1988). Common stressors that contributed to alcohol use included retirement, death of a spouse or close relative, conflict within the family, and physical health problems. Among older adults who suffered alcoholism, stressors were more important contributors to alcohol problems of late onset than early onset.

Alcohol use is associated with many psychiatric disorders (though it is difficult to disentangle which occurs first). The most common disorders that are concurrent with alcohol abuse/dependence are tobacco dependence, organic brain syndrome or dementia, affective or mood disorders, and anxiety disorders. Concomitant drug abuse (usually with prescription drugs) in this study was found among 10 percent of the alcoholics sampled.

Culture may contribute to the onset of alcohol problems as well. Jews, conservative Protestants, and Asians use alcohol less frequently than liberal Protestants and Catholics. Even so, clinicians must be careful to recognize that severe problems with alcohol may emerge in persons from even the most conservative cultural or religious backgrounds with a lifetime history of abstinence from alcohol.

One cultural setting where alcohol use may increase is the emerging affluent retirement community. Only in future years will we better understand the milieu of these retirement communities, for they are constantly evolving. Nevertheless, within this relatively affluent group of older adults with few long-term social attachments who choose to move to an affluent retirement community (either in independent dwellings or in congregate housing), there are persons at risk for alcohol problems. These communities are usually located in warmer and more pleasant climates. One of the more common means of being socially integrated into such a community is to attend the cocktail parties and mixers at the local country club. Persons who have previously been abstinent from alcohol or who have controlled their alcohol intake successfully may find themselves drinking more heavily, given the investment they have made in moving to the community and the anxiety they feel lest they may not be accepted by their peers. Increased unstructured time also contributes to increased alcohol use in such settings.

Results of Alcohol and Drug Use

Alcohol produces significant physical problems for older adults if ingested regularly and in high concentration over time. A major problem is malnutrition, which results from the chronic use of alcohol without proper food intake. Undernutrition usually results in cirrhosis of the liver, one of the eight leading causes of death in older adults. Another problem that accompanies a decrease in liver function is a thinning of the bones (osteomalacia). Chronic alcohol use can lead to a decrease in the ability of the stomach to absorb food and to atrophic gastritis.

Alcohol also affects the brain. Though intelligence may remain intact through many years of heavy drinking, memory tends to decline and the ability to process new information deteriorates remarkably with acute alcohol intake (the intoxication syndrome described above). Together, these physical and cognitive changes associated with alcohol use lead to an increased mortality among alcoholics in mid-life. An alcoholic surviving into late life or older adults who begin to drink heavily in late life often suffer severe physical health problems and cognitive dysfunction.

A further problem resulting from alcohol use is in the interaction between ethanol and other drugs. Sedatives, hypnotics, pain relievers, tranquilizers, and even drugs that relieve motion sickness must be used with caution by people who drink regularly or excessively. Each of these drugs, as well as alcohol, is a depressant of the central nervous system. High doses or combined doses of these drugs can lead to prolonged sleep, failure of respiration, and even death. When alcohol is combined with these drugs, there is a cumulative depressant effect on the central nervous system that renders the older adult impaired in situations that require a quick response, such as driving an automobile or operating machinery like a lawn mower.

Another complication is the physiologic consequences of rapid withdrawal of alcohol. Within a few hours, withdrawal symptoms and signs emerge that reflect the rebound hyperactivity of the nervous system, such as tremors, exaggerated reflexes, and even seizures (delirium tremens). When the older adult suffers malnutrition or physical illness, these rebound symptoms are especially dangerous.

The Diagnostic Workup

The laboratory workup for the older adult who suffers alcohol- or drug-related problems should begin with a measure of blood alcohol or drug level, especially if there are signs of acute intoxication or central nervous system dysfunction. Assays are available for many prescription drugs that tend to be abused by elders. In addition, given the debilitating effects of prolonged alcohol use, it is important to screen blood chemistries, because electrolyte imbalance is common in chronic alcoholics. Liver function studies, especially liver enzymes (LDH, AST, ALT, and alkaline phosphatase), are essential. An electrocardiogram assists the clinician in identifying chronic heart failure, for alcohol can cause muscle damage to the heart and heart failure often leads to rhythm disturbances of the heart.

The diagnostic evaluation of the older alcoholic, however, is most dependent on a thorough history from both the alcoholic elder and family members. Data should be gathered about the type of alcohol consumed by the older adult, how often he or she drinks, whether the drinking is continual or intermittent, and whether the amount of alcohol consumed has increased over time. As guilt and concern about drinking is more frequent in late life compared to other stages of the life cycle, the older person is likely to underestimate the amount of alcohol consumed. Family members should be encouraged to provide accurate information regarding the amount of alcohol the elder has consumed.

Many psychological symptoms accompany acute and chronic alcohol and drug use and should be reviewed in detail. The elder should be asked about symptoms of major depression, generalized anxiety, and suspicious thoughts. Suspiciousness of relatives and friends is frequent among older alcoholics. The presence of suicidal thoughts or impulsive behavior is important to document, given that older white males are at an increased risk for suicide, especially those who live alone and have a history of alcohol use.

Alcohol and drug problems may lead to disruption of sleep in later life. As alcohol is metabolized quickly (as noted earlier), the drug is used by some elders as a sedative, for alcohol produces sedation and sleep initiation. Three to four hours into the night, however, the older adult suffers a rebound from lowering of the blood alcohol level, thus creating significant anxiety and concern about sleeping. Frequently, a benzodiazepine sedative/hypnotic agent is taken at that time, though some elders may take another drink in order to sleep through the remainder of the night.

A thorough evaluation of cognitive functioning, especially memory, is essential. The evaluation is similar to that described in Chapter 2. If, during the office examination evidence of cognitive problems emerges, thorough psychological testing is indicated. If psychological testing is to be of value, however, the clinician must make every effort to test the alcoholic or drug-dependent elder after being abstinent from alcohol or drugs for two to three weeks. When cognitive function during a period of abstinence is normal, these baseline scores can be of value as a reference to document future decline in memory if chronic alcohol use continues.

The physical examination of the alcoholic can be accomplished in large part by observing the elder for signs of chronic alcohol intake. A number of signs suggest chronic alcohol use. Arcus senilis, a ringlike white line encircling the cornea, increases with age and, though it is not associated with a visual disturbance, may also be evidence of chronic alcohol use. Arcus senilis is caused by increased fat in the blood and alcohol increases the concentration of fat in the blood. A red nose (acne rosacea) may suggest the use of alcohol in Caucasians, but many people who are abstinent may have red noses. Cigarette burns, bruises, and cuts should raise suspicion of falls that occur during alcoholic intoxication. An enlarged liver that does not cause the elder any pain suggests alcoholic cirrhosis. Reduced sensation and weakness of the feet and legs occur from nerve damage to the lower extremities, a result of excessive drinking. The physical examination is less revealing of problems involving prescription drug use.

A clinician should interview the family to determine the nature and degree of drug and alcohol use by the elder. The family interview also reveals the degree to which the family is united in their concern regarding the older adult's drug or alcohol problem. As the older alcoholic is likely to resist treatment of any kind, the family must be united if treatment is to be effective. Often one family member may have primary responsibility for some aspect of treatment, such as providing a home for the alcoholic elder during a period following alcohol withdrawal and possibly administering a drug like disulfiram (Antabuse) in order to prevent alcohol use (see page 177). If this family member does not receive support from others in the family (and if the clinician does not recognize this lack of family consensus early in the diagnostic workup), attempts at treating the alcoholic elder are often doomed to failure.

Treatment for Alcohol and Drug Abuse
and Dependence in Late Life

Many of the principles for the treatment of alcohol abuse and dependence in the elderly apply to treatment of elders who abuse the sedative/hypnotic and benzodiazepine drugs. Initial steps in the treatment process are directed to the physical problems that arise during the period of alcohol withdrawal.

When an older adult is evaluated by a clinician and determined to suffer acute alcohol intoxication, the withdrawal process begins. Withdrawal is not only a psychological process, it is a medical process as well—a medical process that may be deceiving. Alcohol tends to dry the mucous membranes and therefore renders the alcoholic elder thirsty. The unwary clinician suspects the older adult is dehydrated and attempts to treat the elder by either encouraging fluid intake or intravenous fluids. It is essential during the diagnostic process to establish the fluid and electrolyte balance, for often the alcoholic is overhydrated. To avoid overhydration, clinicians usually begin by giving a small amount of a hydrating solution (such as 5 percent saline intravenously) while the blood chemistry samples are being analyzed. As alcoholics often subsist on diets high in carbohydrates and low in protein during periods of active drinking, glucose solutions are avoided.

Next, the clinician must prevent the overexcitation of the nervous system that results from the withdrawal of alcohol. Acute problems can be avoided by providing intramuscular injections of magnesium. As magnesium deficiencies are not uncommon in chronic alcoholism and as a decreased magnesium concentration predisposes to the development of seizures and agitation, these precautionary injections are often routine in the treatment of the acute alcoholic. The clinician cannot assume that the older adult will be able to tolerate withdrawal without assistance from a cross-tolerant medication. Cross-tolerant drugs, such as chlordiazepoxide (Librium) and diazepam (Valium), will eliminate the withdrawal effects of alcohol as they replace the pharmacologic effects of alcohol in the nervous system. Therefore one of these drugs should be administered almost immediately and withdrawn gradually over four to five days during the period of acute withdrawal. Alcohol should not be used as a drug of withdrawal. With a cooperative elder and a family who will monitor the dose taken, the elder can undergo withdrawal at home with daily visits to the clinician. Most elders who have a history of chronic use of large amounts of alcohol, however, should be hospitalized for withdrawal.

Following detoxification (the restoration of normal body functionings and the withdrawal of alcohol), older alcoholics usually feel excellent. They promise clinicians and family that they will never touch alcohol again and that they recognize the problems caused by the drug. It is critical to manage this postwithdrawal period effectively when treating the alcoholic elder. Abstinence is the goal, given that the person suffering significant problems with alcohol has already demonstrated an inability to drink occasionally and moderately. One means of encouraging abstinence is the use of disulfiram (Antabuse). Clinicians should prescribe this drug to healthy older adults only, making sure that both patient and family understand the drug's effects. Antabuse dampens the urge to drink, for when alcohol and Antabuse interact in the body, the patient will experience flushing, nausea, and vomiting. The patient "learns" that alcohol use while taking Antabuse is unpleasant, and the habit of chronic alcohol use can be broken more easily.

Self-help groups are most beneficial for support of long-term abstinence from alcohol. Alcoholics Anonymous (AA) has been the most effective of these groups for encouraging abstinence through the life cycle. Alcoholics tend to understand one another better than most clinicians and certainly better than family members. Older persons, unfortunately, often feel uncomfortable with the members of Alcoholics Anonymous (especially if no one their own age or from their own social and cultural background attends). Even so, the chronic older alcoholic should be encouraged to attend these groups. The AA philosophy is usually akin to the values of the older alcoholic, and AA is extremely supportive and perceptive of the needs of the alcoholic, regardless of age. Family members also suffer the consequences of alcoholism and need help from similar groups, such as Al-Anon (a group for family members of alcoholics) and Adult Children of Alcoholics.

Behavior therapy can augment the treatment of alcohol problems. Older adults can learn to relax, to become more assertive, to develop new strategies in socializing with their peers, and to control impulsive behavior through the training and support of a behavior therapist. Many of the positive aspects of AA derive from a behavior therapy approach, for members are given "chips" for successfully abstaining from alcohol for periods of time.

Psychotherapy is of less value in the treatment of alcohol abuse and dependence than was once supposed. Nevertheless, the continued support of the alcoholic elder by the clinician who first treated the individual is essential in the combined therapeutic approach to alcohol.

References

Armor, D., D. Johnston, D. Pollicks, et al. *Trends in U.S. Adult Drinking Practices*. Santa Monica, CA: Rand Corporation, 1977.

Bernadt, M. W., J. Mumford, C. Taylor, et al. "Comparison of questionnaire and laboratory tests in the detection of excessive drinking and alcoholism." *Lancet* 1:325, 1982.

Blazer, D. G. "Alcohol problems in the elderly." In E. W. Busse and D. G. Blazer (Eds.), *Geriatric Psychiatry*. Washington, DC: American Psychiatric Association, 1989. Pp. 489–514.

Blazer, D. G. and M. R. Pennybacker, "Epidemiology of alcoholism in the elderly." In J. T. Hartford and T. J. Samorajskuit (Eds.), *Alcoholism in the Elderly*. New York: Raven Press, 1984. Pp. 25–33.

Blazer, D. G., and I. C. Siegler. "Alcohol abuse and dependence. In D. G. Blazer and I. C. Siegler (Eds.), *A Family Approach to Health Care in the Elderly*. Menlo Park, CA: Addison-Wesley Publishing Co., 1984. Pp. 194–204.

Finlayson, R. E., R. D. Hurt, L. J. Davis, and R. M. Morse. "Alcoholism in elderly persons: A study of the psychiatric and psychosocial features of 216 inpatients." *Mayo Clinic Proceedings*, 63:761, 1988.

Goodwin, D. W., and B. Guzes. *Psychiatric Diagnosis* (4th ed.). New York: Oxford University Press, 1989.

Maddox, G. L., and D. G. Blazer. "Alcohol and aging." *Center Reports on Advances in Research*, 8:4, 1985.

Suggested Reading

Maddox, G., L. N. Robins, and N. Rosenberg (Eds.). *Nature and Extent of Alcohol Problems Among the Elderly* (Research Monograph No. 14). Rockville, MD: NIAAA, 1984.

Mishara, B. L., and R. Kastenbaum. *Alcohol and Old Age*. New York: Grune & Stratton, 1980.

Schuckit, M. A. "Geriatric alcoholism and drug abuse." In *Gerontologist*, 17:168, 1977.

CHAPTER TEN

Emotional Problems Associated with Physical Illness

Physical illness has long been recognized as a major cause of emotional problems in later life and is a frequent companion of the middle-aged and even more of the elderly. As many as 72 percent of persons between the ages of 45 and 64 suffer at least one chronic physical illness. Most of these illnesses are not life threatening nor do they interfere appreciably with the everyday physical and social functioning of the individual. Over the age of 65, 80 percent of the elderly suffer some illness and 50 percent suffer more than one. These illnesses may range from keratoconus, an irregular astigmatism of the eye (which is not easily corrected by glasses and interferes with vision), to chronic retention of urine because of an enlargement of the prostate gland. Neither of these disorders interferes appreciably with normal physical or social functioning. Nevertheless, they are noticed daily and the psychological response to these illnesses can be more disabling than the physical illness itself.

The emotional problems associated with physical illness are of three varieties. Some illnesses produce behavioral symptoms directly. For example, anxiety and hyperactivity are symptoms of increased activation of the thyroid gland in hyperthyroidism. Other illnesses produce symptoms that elicit emotional responses which in turn can make the physical problem worse. For example, the pain and shortness of breath that accompany insufficient blood supply to the heart (angina) may lead to overwhelming anxiety, shortness of breath, and an increased heart rate, which further compromises blood supply to the heart. A third means by which physical illnesses lead to emotional problems derives from complex yet maladaptive thoughts or behaviors generated to adjust to the physical illness.

Most older persons are not seriously ill, nor do they experience significant functional disability. Yet the presence of physical illness in later life increases the risk of emotional problems. If an older adult suffers multiple physical problems, he or she is more likely to suffer severe emotional problems. Severe emotional problems can be found in 10 to 25 percent of hospitalized elderly patients suffering from physical illness (Koening et al., 1988). Less extensive relationships between physical illness and emotional problems are found in outpatient clinics. In a study performed in Monroe County, New York, investigators found that neurotic scores were strongly associated with subjective and objective ratings of physical illness as well as subjective reports of pain and discomfort. In a study of elders in North Carolina, depressive symptoms were found in 64 percent of patients hospitalized for cardiac problems (Dovenmuehle and Verwoerdt, 1962). The following case illustrates the relationship of the physical and emotional problems.

 Mr. Gibson, a successful businessman and the "Don Juan" of the small community in which he lived, was diagnosed at the age of 70 as suffering from cancer of the prostate gland. He had ignored the symptoms of increased difficulty in urination for two years prior to the diagnosis. When he suffered an acute blockage of urination, he was forced to seek consultation in the emergency room, where the cancer was discovered. A team of specialists determined that the cancer had spread to surrounding tissues. Nevertheless, the blockage of urination was severe enough that surgery was required to remove a portion of the prostate gland, which was to be followed by radiation therapy to the surrounding tissues. Surgery was successful and hormone therapy was prescribed (a drug to decrease androgen, the male hormone). The drug prescribed was estrogen, a female hormone. Growth of both the normal and cancerous prostate is dependent on androgens and for this reason estrogen is prescribed to patients suffering prostatic cancer. In addition, both testes of

the patient were removed. Therapy was successful and Mr. Gibson could urinate without difficulty and suffered no pain from the cancer spread to other tissues.

The family of Mr. Gibson was puzzled yet pleased with his response to the therapy. He appeared to have accepted his illness philosophically and seemed more open and concerned about his wife and two children than he had been for many years. He began to make plans for his oldest son to assume responsibility for the family business. He apologized profusely to his wife for the many years of infidelity and, in her presence, asked the forgiveness of God for his sins. The woman with whom he had an affair for ten years was telephoned by Mr. Gibson, the situation explained, and financial support was arranged for her. Mr. Gibson, though he had shown little recent interest in his faith, asked that the Catholic chaplain visit him daily. He confessed his sins repeatedly, noting that he was now being repaid for a lifetime of sin, deceit, and manipulation.

Mr. Gibson also believed it necessary to endure penance for his sin. A lifelong smoker, he forced himself to quit smoking, although the doctors had assured him that quitting would not affect his current condition or prognosis. Withdrawal from tobacco was extremely difficult, and Mr. Gibson often returned to smoking, only to repeatedly quit smoking for a few days, a week, or sometimes a month. He gave large financial gifts to the local Catholic church, gifts so large that the priest contacted Mr. Gibson's physician, expressing concern that he may be acting irrationally. The chaplain attempted to reassure Mr. Gibson that he was having difficulty forgiving himself.

Throughout the early months of diagnosis, surgery, and hormonal therapy for carcinoma of the prostate, the attending surgeon felt it important that Mr. Gibson be seen regularly by a psychiatrist. Mr. Gibson was more than pleased to speak with the consulting psychiatrist, yet did not perceive anything unusual about his lack of concern about his illness coupled with his excessive penance. Four months following surgery, growth of the cancer was identified in x-rays of the bone, yet Mr. Gibson appeared unconcerned.

Mr. Gibson represents one of the reactions to a physical illness, denial, that has been recognized for many years among professionals who work with physically ill older adults. Though he was penitent regarding his past marital infidelity, he made few attempts to reestablish a relationship with his wife, nor did he exhibit a desire to work with her through their joint grieving process. He responded primarily through a denial of his fear of death (though he readily accepted his premature death) and an escape into his faith to the exclusion of his family. He rarely wanted to discuss the illness itself, and, despite the fact that the illness changed his life-style dramatically, he denied the suffering associated with the illness. Rather, he focused on paying his dues, providing for the orderly transfer of his assets to his family, and reestablishing his relationship with God. Mr. Gibson's coping style eventually led to conflict with his family and estrangement from his wife. During the last days of his life, he became acutely depressed, for his family had virtually abandoned him.

Categorizing Emotional Problems
Related to Physical Illness

The categorization of emotional problems that result from physical illness includes both symptoms that result from physical illness and attitudes about physical illness that derive from basic personality structure. Acute and chronic illnesses are, by their very nature, stimuli for some type of emotional response. The symptoms and attitudes described below are abnormal exaggerations of these responses that present special difficulties to professionals working with older adults.

Depression is the most common symptom to derive from physical illness in emotionally disturbed adults. Within the general hospital setting, between 10 and 15 percent of older adults will suffer symptoms of a major depressive episode (see Chapter 4). Another 20 to 30 percent will suffer significant depressive symptoms, though these symptoms are not as easily categorized by the *DSM-II* classification system. Many elders experience adjustment to their illness through depressive symptoms.

Depression may result from certain physical illnesses more than others. For example, depression is frequently a symptom in patients with severe, chronic kidney disease, patients suffering from heart problems (especially those who are recovering from the heart attack or myocardial infarction), and patients suffering from cancer.

The physically ill elderly who have suffered a previous episode of major depression are especially at risk for developing a depressive episode in the midst of a physical illness.

Anxiety is another symptom that often accompanies physical illness in older adults. These elders usually suffer a generalized anxiety disorder (see Chapter 6) rather than panic disorder. The prevalence of anxiety among the physically ill has been reported to be between 20 and 50 percent, though the lower prevalence is probably more accurate. Anxiety disorders are usually less severe than depressive disorders, though the anxious feelings may be especially uncomfortable to the physically ill elder. Anxiety can also interfere with the medical care of the sick older adult.

A third, troublesome symptom is *problems of pain* in physically ill elders. Pain perception may decrease with age and therefore psychogenic pain disorder may be less common in late life than in other stages of the life cycle (there are no good clinical studies to inform us about the relative frequency of problems with pain across the life cycle). Other perceptions decrease as well, such as vision, audition, and touch. Older persons are not as likely to attend pain clinics, even though one of the more common causes of chronic pain—herpes zoster—afflicts 1 to 2 percent of older persons every year. Persistent pain may even increase with age, whereas temporary complaints of pain do not. Temporary pain is defined as pain that is infrequent and not troubling, but which occurs within the two weeks prior to evaluation.

Still another response to physical illness is the *decline in a body function* secondary to the emotional response to physical illness. An example of this mechanism in late life is the decline or cessation in sexual functioning that often follows a heart attack. Though a variety of physical illnesses or insults can lead to impotence in males and decreased sexual enjoyment in females (such as trauma to the pelvic nerve, the use of estrogen hormones in the treatment of cancer, diabetes mellitus, transurethral resection [TUR] of the prostate gland, and drug and alcohol use), many cases of impotence among males and females, especially males, derive from response to psychological stressors or maladaptive psychological reactions to physical illness. Factors such as retirement, a decline in physical health, loss of role, social isolation, lack of a sexual partner, the death of a close friend, or fear following a physical illness contribute to a decrease in sexual drive and a decline in sexual performance. If, for some reason, sexual activity is interrupted for a period of time, such as during an illness, the older adult may be physically capable of returning to full sexual activity, yet because of fears generated by the illness, he or she has difficulty with sexual performance.

Maladaptive Coping Mechanisms in Response to Physical Illness

Clinicians and clinical investigators have characterized many maladaptive attitudes and reactions toward physical illness that derive from particular personality styles. Kahana and Bibring (1964) described seven personality types that are especially useful in understanding the variation in older adults' response to physical illness. Each response can, when exaggerated, decrease the elder's ability to cope with physical illness.

1. *Dependent and overdemanding persons* impress the clinician initially with the urgency of all of their requests. Placing themselves in total submission to the clinician, these individuals are initially optimistic regarding the ability of the clinician to help them, only to become frustrated and angered when their needs are not met. The dependent behavior spreads into other areas, for these persons are at an increased risk for overeating, excessive smoking (even when smoking may prove dangerous to their continued health), alcohol abuse, and abuse of prescription medications, especially antianxiety agents and analgesics.

2. *Orderly and controlled persons* attempt to cast their illnesses in an intellectual light and rely on acquiring as much understanding as possible about the illness. Anxiety is managed through increased understanding of the illness and various therapies. These elders take a ritualistic and often perfectionistic approach to their medical care. They are often orderly, punctual, and extremely conscientious about their medical care. They do not tolerate change and can be most obstinate if unexpected changes or inconveniences occur.

3. *Dramatizing and emotionally involved persons* are traditionally stereotyped as female, though they can just as easily be male. They react to the clinician in a warm and personal way and expect a similar response from the clinician. Sometimes they are teasing and playful, despite the seriousness of their physical disorder. They

display a need to be noticed and admired for their physical appearance. Even while in the hospital, their personal grooming often takes precedence over more important matters. Dramatizing males may attempt to exaggerate their manliness and their sexual prowess with female nurses and physicians. These elders tend to deny their physical illness and become anxious when confronted with the reality of their health problems.

4. *Long-suffering and self-sacrificing persons* regard their difficulties as the result of a lifetime of bad luck. They do not manage their illness well, for they frequently precipitate problems. For example, they tend to be accident prone and will often wait far too long before they seek help, even with minor problems. These persons may allow an ulcer to develop on the lower leg while suffering from diabetes, even though warned frequently by their physician to immediately seek medical attention if they develop a sore on the skin. They almost seem to desire the suffering and to search for punishment.

5. *Guarded and querulous patients* are watchful and suspicious of others, especially medical professionals. They tend to blame physicians and nurses they have seen in the past. As these elders fear the vulnerability that physical illness creates and are naturally suspicious, they view the medical profession and most caregivers as individuals who wish to take advantage of them. Oversights, slights, or hints of negative feelings are interpreted as further evidence that the physically ill elder must be constantly on guard and trust no one.

6. Some elders respond to their illnesses with a paradoxical expression, a *feeling of superiority*. These persons see themselves as all important and influential. Not infrequently, they have achieved some status and therefore are labeled as "VIPs." In response to the threat of physical illness, they maintain a smug, self-centered, or possibly even grandiose attitude. They wish to have only the best physicians and to be hospitalized in only the top medical centers. Even in these centers of excellence, they demand special attention and wish to be treated differently than others. Younger health care professionals are especially at risk for being snubbed or derided by these narcissistic elders. A conflict often arises within these persons, for though they need the care of a competent professional, yet they must maintain superiority over the professional. Such elders argue with professionals regarding the best treatment for the problem or wish to bargain for more control over their care.

7. Some elders appear *uninvolved and aloof.* Mr. Gibson, described earlier in this chapter, is an example of the uninvolved patient. He gave the impression of being remote and reserved and withdrew from everyday concerns within the hospital and at home, even withdrew from the concerns of other people. The aloof elder withdraws into his or her own interests (Mr. Gibson withdrew into religious interests) and does not view emotional ties with others as important, even though he may regret his relations with others in the past. Denial is a means by which elders can protect themselves from the threat of the physical illness.

The Etiology of Emotional Problems Among the Physically Ill

As with other emotional disorders, the causes of emotional problems among the physically ill range from the molecular and cellular to the psychosocial. The number of physical illnesses that can lead to emotional disorders is extensive, including almost all those listed in textbooks of internal medicine. As physical illness precipitates emotional problems in a number of ways, examples of how physical illness can contribute to emotional problems across the biopsychosocial spectrum are presented below.

First, a physical illness can manifest itself directly as an emotional problem recognized for many years. Two examples illustrate this mechanism. First, stroke, caused by damage to brain tissue and manifested by the loss of neurologic functioning (such as paralysis of one side of the body), can cause depression and emotional liability. A stroke in the dominant cerebral hemisphere (usually the left) can cause significant and even severe depressive symptoms, whereas a stroke in a nondominant hemisphere often leads to emotional indifference or even humor and euphoria. The right-handed individual with a left-sided stroke becomes tearful and agitated and exhibits unexpected outbursts of anger many months following the stroke. In contrast, a person with a right-sided stroke often appears indifferent to the severity of the physical disability that has resulted from the stroke. Thyroid dysfunction is also known to contribute to the development of mood disorders. Hypothyroidism, a decreased level of circulating thyroid hormone, produces inactivity, depressed mood, and, when severe, can cause suicide.

A second mechanism by which physical illness precipitates emotional problems is via a maladaptive interpretation of the illness by the older adult. An example from the personality types and their response to physical illness as described by Kahana and Bibring (1964) illustrates this mechanism. In the dependent and demanding elder who suffers a physical illness, the illness is interpreted as a threat to the continuing care from and concern of those around. The elder ultimately fears the final isolation of death. To adapt to this threat of separation, the elder attempts to return, although not consciously, to the secure state of the infant. The dependent older person, therefore, demands unceasing interest and care during the illness. In contrast, the controlled and orderly elder perceives illness as a loss of control. Previous routines are disrupted and previous ordered relationships rearranged. In order to control the anxiety that results from loss of control, these elders intensify their compulsive behavior and become inflexible and opinionated, if not overtly obstinate. Whenever routine is disrupted, such persons exhibit unrealistic and excessive disapproval with those caring for them.

A third mechanism, closely related to the subjective interpretation of the illness, is the impact of the illness upon previous mechanisms for coping. Coping is the means by which each of us evaluates a stressful situation and adapts to that situation. Coping styles vary, depending on personality types and the resultant interpretation of the meaning of a physical illness and the care provided by others associated with that illness. Coping serves at least three purposes. First, coping should decrease the unpleasant feelings associated with a stressful situation, such as a physical illness. In other words, successful coping should decrease anxiety. Second, coping should address the problem itself and its solution. For example, if an elder attends a screening clinic for high blood pressure and learns that his or her blood pressure is dangerously elevated, successful coping would include the acquisition of proper medical care as soon as possible and compliance with that care. Third, coping requires elders to readjust their social relations depending upon the stress, especially if the stress is persistent. If an elder develops severe heart failure, which greatly limits physical activity, then the elder not only must seek proper medical care but must also readjust his activities and substitute new activities for old ones that assure continued life satisfaction.

Impaired coping usually results from exaggerations of personality styles that undermine the adaptation to illness. Impaired coping, such as an overly dependent coping style, may not relieve anxiety but rather exaggerate anxiety. For example, when the elder becomes excessively demanding, health care professionals and family may withdraw. The controlling elder may attempt to cope with high blood pressure by taking on the responsibility for treating the illness. He or she may read about the proper treatment or diet. These attempts to correct the physical problem do not take advantage of medical expertise and endanger the elder's health and physical well-being. Responsibility for care by the elder is useful if not carried to the excess of excluding expert care. The long-suffering and self-sacrificing older adult may cope by resignation to an illness and withdraw from virtually all activities. This behavior disrupts long-standing social relations and interests. Perhaps the elder is not as incapacitated as believed and life expectancy is not decreased because of the illness, yet he or she has instituted a life-style that becomes more problematic over time than the illness.

Another mechanism by which physical illnesses precipitate emotional problems is that they increase stress and the risk for other problems. If a 35-year-old woman breaks her leg in a skiing accident, the disruption of usual activities and inconvenience of the accident can be distressing for a short period of time. Nevertheless, the woman does not experience major disruptions in other areas of her life. Medical insurance covers the cost of the health care, usually a few days to a week in the hospital and outpatient care for the fracture. Disability insurance coupled with the ability to continue portions of her work prevent serious disruption of income and job security. Most middle-aged adults have accumulated enough reserve financial resources that short-term disruptions of work are not major stressors. Family and friends visit frequently and social relations are rarely threatened.

In contrast, older people who suffer hip fractures may immediately find themselves beset with financial problems due to restrictive Medicare payments and confusion regarding copayments from other insurance providers. Their friends cannot visit them in the hospital (transportation and parking are major problems to many elders). They may experience social isolation, though the telephone does provide a means to maintain contact with family and friends. Following discharge from the hospital, their living arrangements may change, especially if they live alone, for they may not be able to care for themselves independently. In other words, a physical illness suffered by an older adult can precipitate a cascade of social and economic problems—multiple vulnerabilities that precipitate emotional problems.

Still another mechanism that contributes to emotional problems associated with physical illness in older adults is the attitudes or beliefs about the physical illness among family, friends, and caregivers. Though illness naturally elicits a sympathetic response, that response is not necessarily empathic. Rather, many family members feel an aversion to contact with the physically ill. This aversion is a vestige of ancient attitudes regarding illness in general. Most fatal illnesses in times past were infectious illnesses. Centuries before the discovery of the "germ" theory of illness, people recognized that there was "something in the air" which could cause an illness. No one could have lived during the times of the bubonic plague (Black Death) and not recognized that association with those who suffered the illness increased the likelihood of developing the illness. Illnesses were contagious and the ill were to be avoided "like the plague."

Attitudes regarding illness were not based upon fact during the time of the Black Death (rats, not people, were the usual vectors of the disease), and today's attitudes are almost as uninformed. In addition, attitudes assert a powerful influence over the behavior of family and friends toward the patient. Though we are well aware that cancer is not caused by contact with someone suffering cancer, there is still something about a cancer patient that drives us away, especially with physical contact. Many illnesses carry a stigma. Older adults suffering an illness soon recognize (if not consciously, at least unconsciously) that family and friends avoid them, especially touching them. Sometimes illnesses can lead to unpleasant odors, cancer being an example. Other illnesses lead to physical deformities, such as changes in the skin, ulcerations, and swelling of body parts. Each of these contributes to the social isolation of the elder suffering a physical illness. Social isolation, then, contributes to anxiety and especially depression. Some elders withdraw further from their social surroundings and devalue themselves, especially their bodies, during an illness. Others attempt to reach out to family more aggressively, only to find themselves even further rejected.

The Diagnostic Workup

Emotional problems that derive from physical illness may result from the direct effect of the illness itself. Therefore, the first step in the diagnostic workup is the medical evaluation of the underlying physical problem. Endocrine and metabolic disturbances, abnormalities of the central nervous system, cancer, intoxication by drugs, or decreased delivery of oxygen to the brain secondary to chronic pulmonary disease each contribute to emotional problems suffered by older adults.

At the level of the organ systems, the evaluation of the functional capacity of the elder adult is essential. To what extent does the physical illness contribute to functional incapacity? For example, why is the elder losing weight? Does the illness interfere with appetite or digestive functions? Perhaps depression has contributed to a decreased appetite. Can the patient eliminate waste products or has the fear of pain upon bowel movement led to excessive constipation? Another elder breathes rapidly. Does lung disease contribute to air hunger and rapid respirations, or is the older adult anxious and therefore is breathing at a faster rate than necessary? Still another elder fears walking in a shopping mall. Is neuromuscular function impaired to the point that mobility is limited, or is the older person fearful or discouraged regarding his or her ability to stand or walk, especially in crowded areas? Many elders fear falling or losing their balance, even when they are perfectly capable of walking. Therefore, they elect to use a walker or a cane and may even request to be transported in a wheelchair.

A complete psychiatric evaluation is as essential as the medical evaluation. The emotional problem, though resulting from the physical illness, may have progressed to a psychiatric disorder requiring the specialized care of the psychiatrist. A mental health specialist should determine if the individual is suffering from a depressive disorder, an organic mood disorder, a panic disorder, or another such disorder. Past psychiatric history and family history must be obtained as well. The risk of suicide must be assessed. The coexistence of depressive symptoms in the medically ill leads to an increased risk of suicide. Poor physical health was a contributing factor to almost half of the suicides committed according to a study by Dorpat and Ripley (1960).

The evaluation of the attitudes and personality styles which contribute to emotional problems in the medically ill requires a more unstructured approach. Though a number of personality inventories are now available (see Chapter 1), personality function and personality disorder is best assessed through an unstructured interview. This interview should take into account not only interaction between the patient and the professional conducting the interview, but should also include an evaluation of interactions between the patient and family and between the patient and professional caregivers. "Typing" of personality—that is, attempting to fit the older adult into the procrustean bed of a specific personality type or disorder—is rarely of value. Rather, the professional determines the degree to which the elder exhibits certain personality traits (see Chapter 1) and in what ways these traits interact with physical illness, as described earlier in this chapter.

An interview with the family should help identify those psychosocial factors that can contribute to the maladaptation of the older adult to the physical illness. The presence or absence of social supports, adjustments in role and changing family roles, and the particular meaning and significance of the illness to both the patient and the family are each important to assess at the outset.

Particular dysfunctions, such as sexual dysfunction, immobility, and incontinence, require special evaluation. Though both the clinician and the patient may be embarrassed to address sexual problems, the loss of the ability to engage in sexual intercourse can be the most disturbing aspect of a physical illness, even more disturbing than its potential to be life threatening. Physicians are in an ideal position to explore sexual dysfunction, for the assessment integrates easily during the diagnostic interview. In addition, the older adult is more likely to inform the physician, especially a primary care physician, of potential problems with sexual performance.

Problems with balance and immobility should be evaluated not only through questions of the patient and his family. The older adult can also be asked to perform neuromuscular tasks in the clinician's office. He can be asked to rise from a sitting position, walk across the office, pick up a moderately heavy object, write his name, and so forth. Dr. Mark Williams at the University of North Carolina in Chapel Hill developed a useful tool for assessing neuromuscular abilities in physical performance (Williams and Jones, 1990). A number of physical tasks are arranged on a board for the older adult to perform. These tasks include placing a latch key into a latch, opening a door knob, turning on a light switch, and adjusting a valve. The assessment of physical functioning is essential to providing sound and useful support to the older adult who is threatened by illness. Even in the midst of a severe illness, function may not be impaired (for instance, during the early and mid stages of cancer). In other situations, functional impairments can be overcome by simple mechanisms that enable the older adult to maintain functional independence. For example, the loss of grip strength may be compensated by having containers in the home that do not require a tight grip in order to open them.

Assessment of incontinence is especially important when evaluating the older woman. Even a well-dressed and intellectually bright elderly woman may experience problems with incontinence. This disorder can require her to wear a pad to prevent soiling her clothes. The sense of loss of control that results from incontinence can be especially threatening to the older woman. The physician or other professional who is not sensitive to this embarrassment and to the potential for overcoming incontinence in older persons who maintain functional independence otherwise may perpetuate emotional problems resulting from incontinence.

Treatment for Emotional Problems
That Result from Physical Illness

Management of emotional problems initially hinges on the management of the physical disorder that underlies the problems. In most cases, the relief of the underlying physical disorder relieves the emotional problem. Nevertheless, in some situations, treatment of the physical problem exacerbates the emotional problem. Aggressive treatment of a cancer may extend life, yet produce pain, discomfort, inconvenience, and financial burden such that the quality of life is minimal to the older adult.

Treatment, therefore, must be "contracted." Physicians and other health care professionals in the nineteenth century were considered "consultants." Opinions were provided and medications prepared. The patient, however, made the final decision regarding the acceptance or rejection of a particular treatment or management program. Modern medicine has become so technologically advanced that the older adult often has difficulty entering into an informed therapeutic contract. Nevertheless, both the health care professional and the elder must never forget the contractual nature of the therapeutic relationship. Active participation by the elder and management decisions that reflect an awareness that the quality of life as well as length of life are important goals ensure that management of the physical illness will improve the emotional well-being of the elder as well.

PHARMACOLOGIC THERAPY

Management of some physical symptoms, such as pain, bridges many illnesses. A number of pharmacologic agents are available to relieve pain. Nonsteroidal anti-inflammatory drugs such as ibuprofen (Motrin, Advil) are now available over the counter. Other drugs, such as naproxen (Naprosyn), must be prescribed. These drugs are especially beneficial for reducing pain that results from inflammatory illnesses such as arthritis. Other analgesics such as morphine are more powerful. These drugs are appropriately used in managing the severe pain following a heart attack.

The successful use of an analgesic has the added advantage of breaking the cycle of chronic pain. The perception of chronic and persistent pain tends to become centralized in the nervous system. When the cause of the pain is treated (possibly through surgery), the pain may persist. Older persons suffering lower back pain may have had a vertebral disc removed (the cause of the pain), yet the pain persists. In some situations, narcotic analgesics, such as meperidine (Demerol), are prescribed for chronic pain. The use of these medications over extended periods can create an even more serious cycle, that of addiction.

The treatment of pain with medications should be augmented by other therapies, for when used in concert, the medications and therapies can provide appropriate pain management. Physical therapy, stress management, appropriate exercises, moist heat, and transcutaneous nerve stimulation are examples of adjunctive therapies. A willingness by the professional to recognize the suffering created by pain and to address pain as a problem, in and of itself, that is to be aggressively and appropriately treated beyond the specific cause (or possibly the original cause) of the pain is essential if emotional problems are to be avoided in the management of chronic pain.

Antidepressant medications are used frequently in the treatment of the chronically ill to alleviate a number of symptoms. Not only are antidepressants prescribed for the treatment of major depression, but they are also used as mild sedatives and in the management of chronic pain.

Some evidence exists that one of the more frequent causes of chronic pain in older adults—shingles, or herpes zoster—is best treated by a combination of a tricyclic antidepressant drug, such as amitriptyline, and a low dose of an antipsychotic agent, such as thioridazine. Yet antidepressant drugs must be used with care in the medically ill because of their frequent side effects. Tricyclic antidepressant drugs:

Increase the likelihood of cardiac rhythm problems

Lower blood pressure, yet interact with some antihypertensive agents, such as alpha-methyldopa (Aldomet), to decrease the effectiveness of these drugs

Increase urinary hesitancy and retention and therefore worsen the inability to urinate with enlargement of the prostate gland

Interact with many drugs that are used in treating physical illness (e.g., may augment the potential of drugs like ephedrine to increase blood pressure or exaggerate the anticholinergic effects of other drugs, such as diphenhydramine (Benadryl)

PSYCHOTHERAPY

Psychotherapy can be used effectively in the treatment of emotional problems resulting from physical illness. Elders who generally resist intervention by a mental health professional often accept the care, support, and interest of a psychiatrist or psychologist who visits daily while the older person is a patient in a hospital or rehabilitation unit. Initial psychotherapy sessions need not be the traditional "fifty-minute hour" but rather may last fifteen to twenty minutes. Psychologists, social workers, and nurses trained in psychotherapy, as well as chaplains and other professionals, can administer psychotherapy in such settings in coordination with the overall treatment goals.

In contrast to the cognitive therapy used to treat the older adults suffering a depressive disorder (see Chapter 4), psychotherapy for the medically ill is most successful when the approach is nondirective and supportive. This approach permits the therapist to gain an understanding of the emotional problems within the context of the physical illness and the life-style of the older adult. Supportive therapy encourages the elder to recognize areas of control in his or her life and contrast those areas to the lack of control he or she has felt during the physical illness. Later in the course of therapy, the elder and the therapist can identify specific areas that need attention.

One such area is that of sexual dysfunction. Therapy can assist the elder in recognizing that the illness does not appreciably interfere with the ability to perform sexually. At other times, therapy may be directed toward assisting the older man or woman in accepting the lack of ability to engage in sexual intercourse, such as following prostatic surgery, within the context of overall sexuality. Specifically, an older man does not lose his identify as a male if he can no longer perform sexually. Spouses are usually supportive, yet the elderly man feels especially threatened when his performance is limited. Intercourse is not the only means by which a couple may express their sexual feelings to each other, and it is not the only means by which they can effect sexual stimulation. Many enjoyable forms of intimacy do not include intercourse, and the therapist can suggest these to the older adult. A positive and carefully developed therapeutic relationship between the elder and the therapist is essential in providing the background for making specific suggestions to the elder for improved sexual functioning.

Personality dysfunction can be addressed therapeutically within the context of the specific personality style exhibited by the physically ill older adult. On many occasions, the strength of particular styles should be emphasized and encouraged. For example, the therapist should acknowledge the elder's wish to be in control, even in the most dependent position in a hospital setting. The therapist should encourage the elder not to "give up" but to take responsibility for his or her own care. The elder and therapist should explore means by which the elder can maintain autonomy and control. For example, some medications may be left at the hospital bedside. The elder can take responsibility for the amount and frequency with which he or she takes the medication, in contrast to giving this responsibility to a nurse. Unfortunately, the medical community's increased concern regarding mistakes in administering medications decreases the patient's autonomy.

Emotional problems that arise in the presence of a physical illness necessarily present a more complex problem to professionals than emotional problems that arise in isolation, even if they are not as serious. Given the complexity of the comorbidity of physical and emotional problems, the art of medicine and mental health care frequently supersedes the science. Few clear therapeutic decisions can be derived from a computer algorithm or decision tree. Yet a humane and balanced approach to care frequently leads to an appreciable improvement in the well-being of the older adult suffering a chronic, even fatal, illness.

References

Dorpat, T. H., and Ripley, H. S. "A study of suicide in the Seattle area." *Comprehensive Psychiatry*, 1:349–359, 1960.

Dovenmuehle, R. H., and A. Verwoerdt. "Physical illness and depressive symptomology: I. Incidence of depressive symptoms in hospitalized cardiac patients." *Journal of the American Geriatric Society*, 10:932, 1962.

Kahana, R. J., and G. L. Bibring. "Personality types in medical management." In Zinberg, E. N. (Ed.), *Psychiatry and Medical Practice in a General Hospital*. New York: International University Press, 1964.

Koenig, H. G., K. G. Meadar, H. J. Cohen, et al. "Self-rated depression scales and screening for major depression in older hospitalized patients with medical illness." *Journal of the American Geriatric Society*, 36:699, 1988.

Williams, N. E., and T. V. Jones. "Predicting functional outcome in older people." In W. R. Hazzard, R. Andres, E. L. Bierman, and J. P. Blass (Eds.), *Principles of Geriatric Medicine and Gerontology* (2nd ed.). New York: McGraw-Hill, 1990. Pp. 1212–1220.

Suggested Reading

Fava, G. A. "The use of antidepressant drugs in the medically ill." In C. Shagass, R. C. Josiassen, W. H. Bridger, et al. (Eds.), *Biological Psychiatry*. New York: Elsevier, 1986. Pp. 583–585.

Hackett, T. P. *Sexual Activity in the Elderly, Clinical Perspectives on Aging*. Philadelphia: Wyeth Laboratories, 1986.

Harkens, S. W., and K. J. Price. "Pain in the elderly." In E. Benedict et al. (Eds.), *Advances in Pain Research and Therapy*, Volume VII. New York: Raven Press, 1984. Pp. 103–121.

Lipowski, Z. J. "Psychiatry of somatic diseases: Epidemiology, pathogenesis, classification." *Comprehensive Psychiatry*, 16:105, 1975.

Rodin, G., and K. Voshart. "Depression in the medically ill: An overview." *American Journal of Psychiatry*, 143:696, 1986.

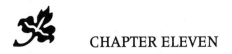

CHAPTER ELEVEN

Bereavement

E*very professional who works with older adults* has encountered the problem of bereavement. At first glance, bereavement would not appear to be an emotional problem. Rather, it seems to be a normal reaction to the inevitable separation from loved ones. Nevertheless, the reactions to separation are varied, and some are pathologic. Those who care for and about older adults can better support them through the grief process if normal grief and its variants are recognized. Grief and depression often coalesce for the professional because the symptoms are so similar. Nevertheless, the normal and pathologic symptoms must be disaggregated. Certain types of treatments to enable coping with pathologic grief, such as an antidepressant drug, should not be used for the treatment of normal grief.

Most professionals learned about the stages of both normal and abnormal grief from Elisabeth Kübler-Ross, whose book *On Death and Dying* received national attention when it was published in 1968. The modern study of the symptoms and management of acute grief, however, began with a classic clinical inquiry by Erich Lindemann in 1945. Dr. Lindemann, a psychiatrist at Harvard Medical School, studied 101 patients who suffered grief reactions, many resulting from the fire in the Coconut Grove nightclub in the early 1940s, where one hundred persons died when they could not escape from the burning building.

In his study, Lindemann recognized that many emotional symptoms that would be abnormal under normal conditions were normal during the stress of bereavement. These symptoms, among others, included bodily distress, such as tightness in the throat, shortness of breath, sighing respirations, and loss of appetite. The bereaved often became preoccupied with the image of the deceased, even seeing the deceased after the death for brief periods of time. Guilt, irritability, and hostility were common symptoms among the bereaved as well. Later, Kübler-Ross suggested five classic stages of bereavement: denial, anger, bargaining, depression, and adjustment.

These reactions to loss occur so often and so regularly that many clinicians have recognized stages of bereavement that occur regardless of age. Do these symptoms occur more often in the elderly? Some investigators suggest that bereavement is more difficult for older adults, as they are more vulnerable to the loss of intimate contact and possible economic hardship that follows a death. The hope of reestablishing a family following the death of a spouse in late life is considerably diminished compared to persons in mid-life. Others, however, suggest that many stressful events, especially bereavement, are better tolerated by the elderly. Bernice Neugarten (1970) described stressful events as being either "off time" or "on time." A 35-year-old woman would be both grieved and surprised at the death of her 37-year-old husband. In contrast, a 75-year-old woman, though she may experience much pain and sorrow at the loss of her 77-year-old husband, nevertheless would have anticipated that she probably would survive her husband. She probably would have rehearsed in her mind how she would adapt to the loss, even if she never discussed it openly. Actually, many older women do discuss openly with their friends the very real possibility that they will survive their husbands and how they will adjust to his death. Whether an older adult adapts better or worse to the loss of a loved one than someone in young adulthood or middle age is of theoretical interest only, for the variation in response, even among the elderly, is considerable. The task of the professional working with the bereaved elder is to meet that elder at the point of his or her unique needs and minister to those needs as best as possible.

As death is a universal human experience, perhaps no emotional problem is more enmeshed in culture than grief. Each culture, and each subculture, has developed both individual and institutional means for coping with this universal human tragedy. In Western cultures, religion is intricately intertwined with the traditions surrounding death. Religious values may, in large part, determine the mode of the disposal of the body (burial or cremation), the nature of the ceremony accompanying the death (a wake or funeral) or, to some extent, the response of the bereaved. For Christians, who believe in a life after death, the death of the loved one is accompanied by the ambivalent feelings of joy that the loved one goes to a more perfect home and sorrow at separation.

At times, religious and cultural norms prevent the persons from experiencing the universal reactions to a loss. Regardless of one's views on what happens to the body, the soul, and spirit on the other side of death, the separation from the deceased, whom we have known on this side of death, is a painful experience. As long as professionals, ranging from the clergy to funeral directors to medical personnel, recognize the need to support the grieving process, even the rituals of funerals can serve the bereaved elder in adjusting to the loss of a loved one.

Bereavement, like other emotional problems, appears to the professional in a variety of guises.

Mr. Taylor, a 72-year-old man, was known to be a difficult patient to all of the doctors who treated him. He suffered a variety of physical problems, including difficulty urinating, back pain, and insomnia. He was also irritable, depressed, and impulsive, which led to a psychiatric consultation. Virtually every member of his family agreed that something had to be done, for Mr. Taylor was a major management problem for both his doctors and his family.

Upon seeing the psychiatrist, Mr. Taylor admitted that he had a number of physical problems. Nevertheless, he had been a strong man most of his life and did not view these problems as being disabling. His major problem was the loss of his prized horse. Mr. Taylor had maintained a small stable of walking horses for many years. He became especially attached to one of these horses, Jenny. Jenny had won a number of prizes at local shows and later in her life had borne more than one colt who had become a champion walking horse as well. When she was sixteen, Jenny had developed an acute intestinal blockage. Mr. Taylor had not been at home at the time, though he returned within a couple of hours after learning of her problem. Even before he returned, he asked his wife to contact the veterinarian, which she did. When the veterinarian arrived, she worked desperately to relieve Jenny of her suffering. Her efforts were to no avail, however, and Jenny died. For the two years following her death, Mr. Taylor blamed himself for her death, repeatedly referring to his neglect of her care. Family members protested that he had lavished more attention on Jenny than he had on his first wife (Betsy) and his current wife.

Betsy had died three years prior to the psychiatric evaluation. Mr. Taylor said very little about her death or his life with her. She had suffered with cancer for approximately six months and had died in a local hospital. Mr. Taylor had remarried about nine months following her death to a woman he had met at his local church some four years previously. Mr. Taylor had been faithful to his wife in the latter part of her life and had no romantic interest in his second wife until after Betsy's death. His sons were resentful, however, that Mr. Taylor had not treated their mother as well as he should. Even on the day of her death, he had delayed visiting her in the hospital because he had been attending to his stable of horses.

After a number of sessions in psychotherapy, Mr. Taylor recognized that his grief over the loss of his prized mare was actually grief over his wife. His overt concern that he had neglected the care of the mare covered his real concern and guilt that he had neglected and abused his wife. When he met and began to date his second wife, within weeks of the death of Betsy, Mr. Taylor had been able to deny his grief. On the death, a year later, of Jenny, the grief broke through, but not in a normal fashion. His bereavement was not directed toward the primary object of his guilt, but displaced, and grief work had not progressed. Bereavement had been prolonged, focused upon physical problems, and had degenerated into a despair about life, despite Mr. Taylor's good physical health and a very supportive and loving second wife.

The Nature of Bereavement

NORMAL BEREAVEMENT

According to the *Diagnostic and Statistical Manual of Mental Disorders* (Third Edition Revised, APA, 1987), persons suffering bereavement may or may not suffer the symptoms of a major depressive episode. Therefore, manifestation of bereavement is similar to clinical depression. There are exceptions to this similarity, however. Uncomplicated bereavement is not associated with a morbid preoccupation with worthlessness, a prolonged and marked functional impairment and significant lack of spontaneity. If guilt is present, the guilt is primarily regarding those things that were done or not done at the time of the loved one's death. If the older adult who grieves normally thinks of his or her own death, these thoughts are limited to thinking that he or she would be better off dead. Suicidal thoughts during normal bereavement are rare. The grief reaction usually does not remain after two or three months.

Grief, however, is not a static phenomenon, but rather a process. Investigators have recognized at least three distinct stages of grief, as recently summarized by Gallagher and Thompson (1989). The first is shock and disbelief associated with feelings of numbness, emptiness, and confusion. Preoccupation with the immediate details surrounding the death predominate. Anxiety is often more prevalent than depression and leads to marked fluctuations in mood during the first few days following the loss of a loved one. Physical symptoms are common, including difficulty with sleep, decreased appetite, and an exaggeration of health problems suffered by the surviving elder. Visits to a physician and requests for medication are therefore common during early bereavement. The "shock phase" is usually pronounced if the death is sudden, unexpected, or unnatural. Such symptoms may even precede the loss of the loved one, or one's own death, when a serious diagnosis is revealed to an older adult and family members.

The second phase of grief emerges as the numbness decreases and depression emerges. Though no "timeline" can be forced upon a grieving elder, this phase usually begins about four to six weeks after the loss. The second phase is not only characterized by a change in the symptoms experienced but is also the time during which friends and families become less available and helpful. The recognition of the finality of the loss coupled with decreased attention from the support network contributes to more crying, chronic disturbance in sleep, decreased energy, fatigue, and withdrawal from usual interests. A desire to be united with the loved one and the preoccupation with the deceased is common during this period.

One aspect of the second phase is the strong sense of the presence and influence of the departed loved one. Actually, this sense of presence can overlap both the first and second phase. If the preoccupation becomes extreme, visual hallucinations of the deceased are not uncommon or abnormal. Occasionally, the bereaved elder hears her name being called or receives mystically a message that all is well. The denial of the death and the sense of unreality about being alone decrease during the second phase, and the true "grief work" begins. Many aspects of the past relationship with the lost loved one are recalled and examined. Unresolved anger toward the loved one, perceived neglects, and subsequent guilt emerge and a search for an explanation as to the reason for the death becomes another preoccupation.

This phase of bereavement generally persists at least a year, usually through the first anniversary of the death of the loved one. The first nadir of grief often occurs approximately one month after the loss, and a second nadir occurs approximately six months after the loss. Most students of bereavement report a noticeable improvement in outlook and a reduction in dysfunction after six months, though each "anniversary" can precipitate recurrences of the symptoms that characterize the second phase. Anniversaries, not only of the death but also birthdays, wedding anniversaries, special holidays, and planned events that were never carried out become difficult times, especially during the first year of grief.

The third phase, which usually predominates after the first year, is resolution of the grief process. This phase has been variously labeled acceptance, identity reconstruction, and reintegration. The bereaved elder begins to initiate new social contacts and to reorganize her life around activities and interests that do not involve the lost loved one. Though brief periods of acute depression recur, with crying and a return of the feelings of emptiness, they are less frequent and lead to fewer morbid thoughts. Physical symptoms such as sleep loss, decreased appetite, and loss of energy disappear. Past events are recalled with pleasure and the elder welcomes opportunities to talk about the lost loved one with others. The acceptance phase requires at least another year before relative normality returns and a new lifestyle is established.

Some professionals expect the bereaved elder to march step systematically through these phases. This is a misconception. Though grief usually requires about two years to progress to completion, there is much variation around the two-year average. The time required for bereavement is determined by the emotional resources of the individuals and the circumstances of the death. Some individuals grieve effectively over a six-month period. A new marriage nine months after the loss of a spouse of fifty years in this situation is not abnormal. Others suffer significant hardships and pain for four to five years, yet the work through grief progresses and eventually resolves.

A second misconception regarding grief is that these phases follow one another sequentially. The shock, disbelief, and anger that initially accompany grief can recur throughout the grief process. For example, a bereaved older adult may become angry and suspicious for no obvious reason one year after the death of a loved one. When explored, the anger relates specifically to the bereavement, and therefore can be addressed in counseling.

Zisook and Shuchter (1986) studied bereaved men and women over a four-year period. They found the most severe, effective, and symptomatic distress occurring during the first month following the loss of a loved one. Anger and guilt were frequent symptoms, especially during the first months. Yet anger in persons who believe themselves to be responsible for a spouse's death was found to be more enduring than guilt. Depression persisted throughout the four years, though the symptoms of depression became less severe with time. After the first year of bereavement most of these widows and widowers believed they could function as effectively as before the death. Social involvement increased dramatically after the first anniversary of the death. In contrast, the ability to enjoy sexual relations remained stable during the first year of grief and increased thereafter. Nearly 50 percent of the bereaved stated that they still enjoyed sex one month following the loss of a loved one. One-fourth of the bereaved were remarried the fourth year following the death of a spouse.

ABNORMAL BEREAVEMENT

The vicissitudes of abnormal bereavement are legion. Nevertheless, abnormal grief is an emotional problem that professionals working with elders must recognize and which requires professional intervention. The first of these abnormal grief reactions is *delayed grief*. Though a slight delay may be normal, for the older adult may be preoccupied with the events surrounding the death, delay of grief for weeks and months is abnormal. Unfortunately, these elders are often praised by the family and community for adjusting so well to the loss. "He hardly shed a tear at the funeral and is going right along with his life." Yet when grief is postponed, a price is paid. These individuals often experience a sudden and unexpected onset of symptoms, often around anniversaries (such as birthdays and special holidays). Other persons who delay their grief enter a detached numbness during which they deny virtually all emotional reaction to not only the loss but also other events in their lives, such as changing financial status and changing roles. These persons withdraw from others or they mask their emotional symptoms with physical problems and beleaguer their primary care physicians. Another abnormal delay results from a denial of the reality of the loss. Such delayed grief may result from an unnatural death, for example, if the body was mutilated or destroyed.

Response to an unnatural death presents a more complicated problem to the professional working with the bereaved elder than a death from natural causes. Unnatural deaths include volitional deaths—such as from homicide or suicide—and accidental deaths, such as automobile accidents, drowning, falls, or natural disasters (Rynearson, 1986). The usual response to an unnatural death includes symptoms not generally associated with bereavement as well as the normal symptoms of bereavement. Hyperactivity, startle reactions, intrusive recollections of the trauma (even though the elder did not witness the event), and a blunting of feelings often accompany an unnatural death. Other survivors experience a sense of victimization. If an elderly man is robbed and murdered while returning home from grocery shopping, his bereaved wife may believe the death an unforgivable act and may experience great difficulty in resolving the anger regarding the death. Vengeance may dominate her life for months, even years. Still other elders who experience the loss of a loved one by an unnatural death, such as homicide, may develop an existential anxiety. If a loved one can be taken so unexpectedly, can there be any protection from the inhumanity of one person toward another?

The reaction of a family to death following a suicide is especially difficult. Anger toward the loved one is common and is associated with severe guilt, for most family members believe they could and should have recognized the danger signs and therefore prevented the death. Families must also adapt to the embarrassment of the suicide, especially if it was well publicized. Family members who are deeply religious may believe that the suicide victim automatically goes to eternal punishment with no chance of redemption. Despair, frustration, and a feeling of helplessness predominate the feelings of the individual suffering bereavement from a suicide.

Prolonged or unresolved grief is another abnormal variant of the grieving process. A number of symptoms are associated with the complicated, unresolved grief, especially excessive guilt regarding the circumstances of the loss or anger toward persons who are associated with the death, such as health care professionals. If the process of grief does not move toward resolution, other problems arise, such as the precipitation of a major or clinical depressive episode and decline in physical health, which may result in accelerated mortality for the surviving elder. Prolonged grief often can be predicted early in the grieving process, especially if the older adult has not adapted well after the first month or two following the loss. The experience of additional social stressors (such as problems with children), economic hardship, and a history of emotional problems prior to the death of the loved one also predict a poor outcome.

Distorted variants of normal symptoms should alert the professional to abnormal bereavement. Goldfarb (1974) described one variant as *pseudoanhedonia*. Bereaved elders act and speak as if to say, "I'm without feeling and nothing matters. Do whatever you want with me." Not only are they denying appropriate response to the loss, they deny other feelings as well. Such elders insist upon being left alone—not being pushed into activities—and appear as martyrs. This lack of feeling and apathy may be an unconscious means of punishing themselves or another. Though such behavior can elicit sympathy, or possibly admiration, from the social network, the ultimate result is detachment from others.

Another abnormal symptom of grief is *increased activity without a sense of loss*. The bereaved elder behaves virtually opposite to what others expect. He or she exhibits a zest for activities, may become adventuresome when previously reserved, and makes rash decisions. Still another abnormal response is *taking on the symptoms of the person who has died*. These elders often believe they suffer from the same disorder that killed their loved one, perhaps a cancer or a heart attack, and persistently seek medical attention for imagined ailments that mimic ailments suffered by the deceased prior to death. Professionals must be careful not to dismiss these complaints out of hand, for the increased mortality of a surviving spouse can be prevented if appropriate medical intervention is instituted.

Another abnormal reaction is *hostility*. The elder may be especially angry at a physician who was caring for the spouse at the time of death. She may accuse him of neglecting his duty or even willful behavior that hastened the death of the loved one. Though most elders do not act upon these hostile feelings (such as filing a malpractice suit), prolonged anger does complicate the resolution of the grief process.

Social isolation is still another abnormal reaction and one that can be especially problematic. The bereaved elder has difficulty initiating any social activity and shows little response to those who wish to engage him in new or even previous activities of interest. After a while, family and friends attempt contact less frequently and the elder becomes progressively more isolated. A vicious cycle emerges. Even if a friend contacts the bereaved elder in an attempt to break the cycle, the elder interprets this as not a true demonstration of friendship but rather an obligation. He may even feel denigrated by the request to join a friend for a meal or attend a social gathering. Social isolation contributes to increased suspiciousness and paranoid thoughts in a bereaved elder, similar to those described in Chapter 5 on suspiciousness and agitation.

The Etiology of the Grief Reaction

The origin of the grief reaction appears deeply embedded in the human spirit. Even primates exhibit behavioral responses that mimic the grief process. Though an unwillingness to develop attachments to others can be devastating to a person throughout life, the loss of firmly established social attachments leads to biologic and psychological responses that are predictable and easily measured. McKinney (1986) reviewed the relevance of primate separation studies to bereavement. When certain species of monkeys are separated from their parents, beginning virtually with the first night of separation, both heart rate and body temperature are decreased. If the young monkey is returned to the parent the next day, the heart rate and body temperature return to normal. If the time until a return is prolonged, however, permanent changes occur.

In a separate study among a different species of monkeys, maternal separation led to significant elevations in plasma cortisol, similar to the elevation of plasma cortisol described among the more severe depressions in humans. Kosten et al. (1984) studied thirteen older adults who had suffered an acute loss within six months prior to the study. These persons met criteria for major depressive disorder symptoms considered normal during the grief process. These investigators found that cortisol levels following administration of dexamethasone, which should be lowered, were higher than would be expected but were not as high as found in individuals suffering from major depression (see Chapter 4). The cortisol levels were correlated with the severity of the depressive symptoms. Therefore, severe depressive symptoms during grief can lead to abnormalities in the endocrine system, though not as severe as found in major depression.

Other investigators, especially Harry Harlow (1971), have described the psychological response of young animals separated from their mothers. Virtually all such investigators have identified behaviors that have been labeled "protest" and "despair." During the protest stage, the young animals appear agitated, emit distressed vocalizations, and exhibit increased oral behavior, such as feeding and touching the lips. This stage is followed by the despair or depressed stage, which is characterized by a decrease in activity, huddling in the corner of a cage, and general social withdrawal.

Because adult animals, for the most part, do not exhibit firm and lasting attachments, except females toward their infants, it is difficult to equate such studies except in the recognized attachment of mothers to their infants among primates. Nevertheless, the grief reaction appears innate from birth and inherent among all primates. The many variations on this basic theme, both normal and abnormal, derive from the psychological makeup, the physical health, and the social/environmental context in which bereavement progresses.

The Diagnostic Workup

The evaluation of the bereaved elder derives directly from an understanding of the spectrum of bereavement and the context in which bereavement occurs. Unlike other emotional problems suffered by the elderly and described in this book, there is no specific approach to evaluating the bereaved. Rather, the professional must first become acquainted with the bereaved elder and the circumstances of the loss.

- What was the previous physical and emotional health of the bereaved elder?
- Was the death natural or unnatural?
- Was the death expected or unexpected?
- Have additional stressors complicated bereavement beyond what is normally expected?
- Are the symptoms experienced by the bereaved elder, given the time since the loss, appropriate to the magnitude of the loss?
- Has the process of grieving followed a normal course of bereavement?
- What has been the response of family and friends to the bereaved elder?
- Do family and friends view the response of the bereaved elder to be normal or abnormal?

In addition, the professional must especially attend to the physical health of the bereaved elder.

- Has the elder maintained adequate dietary intake, physical exercise, and personal hygiene?
- Are there signs of emerging physical problems, such as cardiovascular disease?
- Has the elder continued to take medications that were prescribed for physical problems dating from before the bereavement?
- Does the elder maintain appropriate health habits? For example, an elder suffering from chronic lung disease, who stopped smoking many years prior to the bereavement, may return to smoking as a means of reducing anxiety.

In the evaluation of the bereaved older adult, the basic goal should be to identify particular risks for abnormal bereavement, psychiatric illness, and/or physical illness. An important caveat should be remembered by the professional working with bereaved elders: Males usually experience more difficulty with bereavement than females. There are a number of reasons for the increased problems among males in the latter part of the twentieth century (though this may change in the twenty-first century with a new cohort of men who practice different life-styles than the current cohort of elderly males). For one, men are less likely to lose a spouse than are women. The bereaved man is therefore not as prepared to live alone as is a widow. In addition, return from the office to home and retirement may be associated with difficulties in adjusting, for men often do not know "what to do around the house." If a spouse dies, then the man does not feel comfortable in the home.

Men also are frequently less adept in the many practical tasks which must be accomplished around the house, tasks that have traditionally been considered "female" tasks. These tasks include cooking, cleaning, shopping, laundry, and even managing a household budget. Faced with such new tasks, men are less likely to seek help from others, for they wish to sustain an image of self-sufficiency during bereavement.

Men are at greater risk because they are likely to be more restricted in expressing their feelings. Women tend to maintain a number of close friends to whom they can speak of their deepest feelings. Men, in contrast, have many social acquaintances but few, if any, friends with whom they can share their deepest thoughts and feelings. Emotional isolation becomes severely exacerbated at the loss of the spouse.

Men may also be "surprised" at the loss of a spouse. As noted above, bereavement for women usually is an expected event, that is, they expect to survive their spouse and have rehearsed what their lives might be following the death of their husbands. In contrast, men expect to die before their spouse, if they think about death at all. Therefore, they do not consider life apart from their wives and the death of a spouse becomes especially traumatic.

There are many gaps in our knowledge regarding the differential effects of bereavement between men and women. Generalization rarely applies totally to an individual. Nevertheless, the professional must be aware that men are especially at risk for problems during bereavement, and therefore close monitoring of the bereaved elderly male is essential (Feinson, 1983).

The evaluation of the bereaved elder should also include an evaluation of the support network of that elder. A review of objective and subjective support during the weeks that immediately follow bereavement is not usually an accurate reflection of persistent support. Nevertheless, after two to three months, trends emerge that may indicate to the professional particular risks to the bereaved elder. For example, how many persons are available to the bereaved older adult? One means by which this can be determined is to select a series of normal needs that might be requested of family, friends, and acquaintances. These needs may range from the availability of someone to check one's house or apartment and feed one's pet for a two- or three-day vacation to the availability of a friend or acquaintance to whom the older adult can talk about his or her deepest and most troublesome concerns. The social network will range from family to friends to professionals. For example, a relatively isolated elder may develop a relationship with her physician and therefore can share with the physician virtually anything about her life.

- How often does the elder interact with the social network? For example, how many phone calls are made during the day and how many calls are received?
- Does the elder go out almost every day? If so, are the trips visits to someone else?
- Does the elder belong to regular activities, such as religious groups or clubs?
- Does the elder maintain an active correspondence with family and friends?
- If the older person wishes to vacation, does he or she have family or friends with whom vacationing is likely?

Next, the social network should be evaluated for its perceived value to the bereaved elder.

- Does the elder believe that he or she still belongs to and fits into the family and the community?
- Does the bereaved elder understand the activities that take place around him or her? For example, does an elderly man who has attended a synagogue for most of his life still recognize and feel comfortable with the procedures and activities of the synagogue?

- Does the older person feel that he or she is understood by others? If hearing and visual impairments are moderately severe, these communicative abilities may decrease, leading to further social isolation.

Most elders have at least one intimate relationship, as do most people throughout their life cycle. Bereavement, however, may disrupt that one intimate relationship and place the elder at specific risk for social isolation.

Finally, it is essential to determine if persons are available to the bereaved elder to perform specific tasks that may be needed, even if needed temporarily. Are there persons to cook meals, assist in cleaning the house, or assist with the financial arrangements following the death? Is someone available to stay with the bereaved elder for a short period of time, or can the elder move for a time to the home of a child?

Treatment for Bereavement in Late Life

The goal of successful counseling and support of the grieving older adult is straightforward—facilitate normal grief. If the elder grieves normally and appropriately, progress toward resolution and adaptation to life without the lost loved one will be forthcoming. In counseling the bereaved, therefore, encouraging the elder to "work" in those areas that have been neglected is the most helpful approach to therapy. Grieving can begin before the loss. For example, as the personality of a spouse deteriorates with the progression of Alzheimer's disease or a fatal physical illness reaches its final stages, the grieving process usually begins before death and may be largely completed at the time of death.

PREPARING AN ELDER FOR A LOVED ONE'S DEATH

A recognition that grief can begin even before death underlies the importance, not only to the dying older adult but to the family as well, of humane and dignified care through the process of dying. The development of hospice services (founded by Cicily Saunders) represents a means by which the dying receive humane but not aggressive medical care. Pain and suffering are relieved to the maximum yet the process of dying is not unnaturally prolonged through aggressive interventions. Not every elder, or indeed every family, will choose to participate in hospice programs. Nevertheless, such options should be available to older adults and their families. Hospice teams usually consist of physicians, nurses, mental health professionals, and clergy. Family support is at least as important in caring for the dying patient as support of the older adult herself.

Another step to facilitate coping with bereavement is to assist the elder who is caring for a dying loved one to communicate with that loved one (Lucas and Siegler, 1984). Encourage the elder to spend time with the dying person and not to avoid interaction. Encourage the elder to listen attentively to the dying and give the attention that is necessary. Interaction should be tactful and honest. There are no "right and wrong" things to say. Being there is of greater importance than stumbling upon the right words to say.

HELPING THE ELDER THROUGH THE EARLY STAGES OF BEREAVEMENT

Once death occurs, the first step to be taken in caring for the bereaved elder is to intervene by dampening the crisis of the bereavement (Rabin and Pate, 1981). The elder will remember vividly those circumstances under which he or she receives news of the death of the loved one. She often will recall the tone, the context, and the inflection used by the person who tells her of the death. The news of death should usually be imparted by that physician primarily responsible for the care of the deceased prior to death, or by a close friend of the family. If the information is delivered by a stranger, then some suspicion of malpractice or secrecy ensues. The elder can be prepared for the tragic news by statements such as, "Let's sit down and talk together. I have something to tell you." This appears to be prolonging the inevitable: nevertheless, it breaks the news gently. If a fatally ill loved one is being resuscitated and the resuscitation appears to be ineffective, the physician or staff should inform the family of the crisis and that things "do not look good."

Once the elder is prepared for the tragic news, it is best to be clear and concise regarding the news. Then the physician should be available to the bereaved elder to answer any questions and to ensure support of the bereaved during the period of acute crisis.

Medications should be used only in the most severe circumstances. Anxiety, depression, and lack of sleep are to be expected during the acute phases of grief. On the other hand, if the surviving spouse has spent many days suffering broken sleep, a mild sedative, such as hydroxyzine (Vistearil) or diphenhydramine (Benadryl), can be given to assist sleep and readjust the sleep-awake cycle. Minor tranquilizers (antianxiety agents), such as diazepam (Valium), should be used judiciously but may be necessary for a few days during the acute phase of grief.

Once the older adult progresses through the acute phases, supportive psychotherapy may be needed to facilitate normal grieving. A number of guidelines for these supportive therapies can assist clinicians working with the bereaved elder (Blazer, 1982). First, the therapist should permit and help the older adult to put into words and nonverbal expressions the pain, sorrow, and the finality of the loss. A review of the relationship with the deceased is most important in this process, that is, a life history approach. The bereaved may even be asked to write down instances, both good and bad, of interaction or shared experiences with the lost loved one.

The bereaved elder should be encouraged to discuss the feelings of love, guilt, and especially hostility toward the deceased, for anger is often the last emotion to be expressed but yet may be the most important emotion to discuss. The bereaved elder should be helped to recognize changes in thoughts, feelings, and behaviors that are associated with bereavement and not to imagine himself or herself abnormal. Education regarding grief can be most helpful. A number of excellent books have been written describing the grieving process. Encouraging the use of these books places the feelings of the elder in context.

Therapists should avoid interpreting long-standing conflicts between the bereaved and the deceased during the period immediately following the loss. Long-term reintegration of thoughts, especially when there may have been infidelity on the part of the lost loved one, poor financial management, or physical abuse, will complicate the grief process initially. In time, however, these conflicts must be addressed if they cannot be resolved spontaneously by the bereaved elder.

Most persons bring their own unique strengths to the grieving process. These strengths should be supported. For example, some denial and activity may be the best means by which an older adult can negotiate bereavement effectively. The bereaved should be reassured that the suffering and pain are transient. If the bereaved becomes inordinately attached to the professional, these transference reactions should be permitted and dependency of the bereaved on the professional (i.e., a transition object) for a period of time can be most beneficial. In time, sessions with the bereaved can be decreased, but abrupt terminations of professional contact, reminiscent of the death, should be avoided.

SELF-HELP PROGRAMS

There are many self-help programs for assisting the elder in coping with bereavement. Widow-to-widow programs that provide peer counseling and support during the months immediately following the death can be of great importance to the older adult. As with alcoholism, bereavement is best understood by someone who has also undergone a similar experience. For those persons who have progressed further in the grieving process, the ability to reach out and help others has a therapeutic benefit to the helper. A sense that the bereaved elder is not alone is essential for successful grieving.

The therapist and other professionals working with the bereaved elder should work ultimately toward facilitating reintegration into the world. The elder should be judiciously counseled regarding the development of new relationships and changes in lifestyle. Nevertheless, the bereaved elder should also be cautioned regarding the development of sudden attachments that may result from a desire to substitute another person for the lost loved one. Counseling around these issues can be especially beneficial in facilitating the universal experience of bereavement.

References

American Psychological Association. *Diagnostic and Statistical Manual of Mental Disorders* (3d ed.). Washington, DC: American Psychological Association, 1987.

Blazer, D. "Late life bereavement and depressive neuroses." In D. Blazer (Ed.), *Depression in Late Life*. St. Louis: C. V. Mosby, 1982. Pp. 164–177.

Feinson, M. C. "Aging widows and widowers: Does the impact of bereavement differ?" Paper presented at the Gerontological Society of America annual meeting, November 1983.

Gallagher, D., and L. W. Thompson. "Bereavement and adjustment disorders." In E. W. Busse and D. G. Blazer (Eds.), *Geriatric Psychiatry*. Washington, DC: American Psychiatric Press, 1989. Pp. 459–473.

Goldfarb, A. I. "Minor maladjustments of the aged." In S. Arietis (Ed.), *American Handbook of Psychiatry*, Volume I. New York: Basic Books, 1974. Pp. 820–860.

Harlow, H. F., and Suomi, S. J. "Production of depressive behaviors in young monkeys." *J. Autism and Childhood Schizophrenia*, 1:246–263, 1971.

Kosten, T. R., S. Jacobs, and J. W. Mason. "The dexamethasone suppression test during bereavement." *The Journal of Nervous and Mental Disease*, 172:359, 1984.

Kübler-Ross, E. *On Death and Dying*. New York: Macmillan, 1969.

Lindemann, E. "Symptomology and management of grief." *American Journal of Psychiatry*, 101:141, 1945.

Lucas, R. A., and I. C. Siegler. "Death and dying." In D. G. Blazer and I. C. Siegler (Eds.), *A Family Approach to Health Care in the Elderly*. Menlo Park, CA: Addison-Wesley, 1984. Pp. 222–225.

McKinney, W. T. "Primate separation studies: Reference to bereavement." *Psychiatric Annals*, 16:281, 1986.

Neugarten, B. L. "Adaptation and the life cycle." *Journal of Geriatric Psychology*, 4:71, 1970.

Rabin, P. I., and J. K. Pate. "Acute grief." *Southern Medical Journal*, 74:1468, 1981.

Rynearson, E. K. "Psychological effects of unnatural dying on bereavement." *Psychiatric Annals*, 16:272, 1986.

Zisook, S., and S. R. Schuchter. "The first four years of widowhood." *Psychiatric Annals*, 16:288, 1986.

Suggested Reading

Brown, J. T., and A. Stoudemire. "Normal and pathological grief." *Journal of the American Medical Association*, 250:378, 1983.

CHAPTER TWELVE

Working with the Family of the Older Adult Suffering Emotional Problems

Older adults do not cope with emotional problems in isolation. Rather, they cope with others who provide social and emotional support in a milieu that provides a sense of connectedness and belonging (Atchley, 1985). Though many older adults (especially women) are no longer married and do not live with other family members, families remain the most important source of social and emotional support for older adults in Western society. Therefore, professionals working with older adults suffering emotional problems must understand the older adult in the context of the family and facilitate coping, at least in part, through the family.

Who is part of the family of the older adult? Family can be individuals who are genetically related or who have developed relationships and/or are living together as if they were related (Miller and Miller, 1979). The concepts of "nuclear family" and "extended family" have taken on increasing relevance in recent years due to the mobility of Western society. The nuclear family includes husband, wife, and children, all of whom usually live in the same household. Extended family consists of other relatives, such as parents, grandparents, siblings, aunts, uncles, and cousins. To work effectively with the older adult, the professional must include both the nuclear and the extended family in therapy, although the actual number of family members contacted is usually limited.

Families are best understood as a living system (Miller and Miller, 1979). A system, according to general systems theory, is a set of units or nodes with relationships among them. The state and trait of each node is influenced by other nodes in the system. Though relationships with other nodes do not determine all characteristics of node (for example, the feelings or behavior of the older adult), they do shape behavior to a considerable extent. Systems theory is complex, however, and therapies derived from systems analyses are not that much more practical than therapies derived from general intuition about human relations. Nevertheless, professionals must never ignore the importance of human relations when attending the emotional problems presented by the older adult. Problems throughout this book have been described as "individual" problems, such as the older adult who must cope with the problem of depression. Individual, however, does not mean autonomous. The following example illustrates the relationship of family members and elders with emotional problems.

 Mr. and Mrs. Faulkner were 68 and 65 years of age, respectively, when they decided to move from Chicago to a rural community in North Carolina to be near their 45-year-old divorced daughter, Mary. Mary had struggled financially to raise her children for years after divorcing her husband. Mary's children had completed school and had obtained work locally, and she welcomed her independence, enjoying her work as a librarian at the local high school. She was therefore surprised when her parents announced their intentions to move.

Mary and her parents had maintained an excellent relationship throughout her life. Her mother had been a tremendous support to her during the time that she was adjusting to the separation and divorce from her husband. She welcomed her parents to the small North Carolina community and her parents, always independent, provided companionship for Mary without interfering with her life-style.

Five years after moving to North Carolina, Mrs. Faulkner began to suffer difficulty with her memory. She could no longer prepare meals, she became lost on more than one occasion while driving to visit friends, and was progressively withdrawing from social activities that she previously shared with Mr. Faulkner. At the insistence of Mary, Mr. Faulkner sought the consultation of a local doctor regarding the memory problems. Mrs. Faulkner was suffering from primary degenerative dementia of the Alzheimer's type (Alzheimer's disease) and the condition had progressed significantly. Only the attentive care of Mr. Faulkner had permitted Mrs. Faulkner to continue to maintain an independent life during a rapid decline in her memory. Mary was concerned that her parents could no longer care for themselves (for her father had never been helpful around the house). She was surprised that her father had been able to rise to the occasion and take over many household responsibilities. His dedication to Mrs. Faulkner was admired by Mary and others who were acquainted with the family.

The year following the diagnosis of Alzheimer's disease, Mr. Faulkner began to suffer chest pain and shortness of breath. Because he was so busy caring for his wife, he neglected seeking medical care until encouraged by Mary. Mr. Faulkner was referred to a specialist after initial evaluation by his local physician. A chest x-ray and biopsy confirmed the worst of Mary's fears. Mr. Faulkner was suffering from a rapidly spreading cancer of the lung. The disease had progressed to the point that surgery was impossible. Radiation therapy and chemotherapy were thought to be of some benefit.

Mr. Faulkner underwent a course of radiation therapy from which he became very weak and discouraged. He no longer could perform household chores nor could he prepare meals. Mrs. Faulkner seemed unaware and unconcerned about the change in Mr. Faulkner's physical health. Mary decided that a live-in housekeeper was the only solution. She searched throughout the small town for three weeks and finally identified a woman who appeared ideal for the task. She was able to recruit the woman with an excellent salary (for the Faulkner family had acquired considerable financial resources). For two weeks, the live-in housekeeper cared for Mr. Faulkner during his convalescence and worked well with Mrs. Faulkner. Unfortunately, Mrs. Faulkner did not understand why this "other woman" was in the house. She accused her husband and the woman of having an affair. When she elevated the intensity of her complaints, the housekeeper could no longer tolerate Mrs. Faulkner's badgering and left.

Mary, once again, searched for a housekeeper. After two additional recruitments of responsible persons in the home, each left because of the badgering of Mrs. Faulkner. During this period, however, Mr. Faulkner regained his strength. For the next four months, he was able to resume most of the household chores. Mary visited her parents every day and assisted with housework and meal preparation approximately an hour each day.

Mr. Faulkner's condition again deteriorated and he was forced to return to the hospital for a second course of radiation therapy. Mary moved her mother to her own home during the hospitalization, but this move became stressful for both Mary and her mother. Despite her mother's memory difficulties, old conflicts regarding control between Mary and her mother emerged. Mary, in turn, sought another housekeeper to stay with her mother while her father was in the hospital. Mr. Faulkner's condition did not improve, and he did not return home but was discharged from the hospital to a nursing care facility. Mrs. Faulkner exhibited no understanding of Mr. Faulkner's condition nor the change in living arrangements, even though she visited her husband every other day.

Mary faced another crisis. She could not care for her mother alone, her mother did not appear to be "ill enough" to be admitted to a nursing care facility herself, yet her mother would not allow anyone to care for her in her own home because of her confusion regarding the role of the person in the home with her. Mary discussed these problems with her mother's physician as well as a social worker. It was decided that the most appropriate intervention was to admit Mrs. Faulkner to the same nursing home with her husband. Mrs. Faulkner did not protest this move and seemed to adjust relatively well. Most of the time, she was unaware that her husband was in the same nursing home, even though she would go to his room and visit four or five times a day. Though he was in great pain and suffered much during the terminal stages of cancer, he maintained an understanding of his wife's confusion and lack of empathy and supported his daughter Mary in her decision. Three months after Mr. Faulkner was admitted to the nursing home, he died. Mrs. Faulkner continued to reside in the nursing home for three years and was visited two or three times a week by her daughter. After the first year, Mary was unsure that Mrs. Faulkner even knew who she was.

In this complex example of the memory problem suffered by Mrs. Faulkner, appropriate care could not be provided without recognizing the family interactions, stresses on the individual family members, and the resources available to these family members to provide care for Mrs. Faulkner. Though only three family members were of importance in the care of Mrs. Faulkner, their interrelationships and the recognition of the needs of each was more essential for humane care of not only Mrs. Faulkner but Mr. Faulkner and Mary.

Problems Faced by Families of Older Adults with Emotional Problems

THE IMPACT ON THE CAREGIVER

One of the more common problems facing families is the burden placed upon caregivers of persons suffering from chronic illnesses in late life, especially primary degenerative dementia. The debilitating course of dementia coupled with as yet poorly developed community and professional support services place responsibility for care predominantly on families until the later stages of the disease. A number of problems may result from the time and effort required to care for a debilitated elder, such as anger, guilt, self-pity, and depression. Not only can the responsibilities of caregiving precipitate emotional problems in other family members, these burdens disrupt well functioning family systems that provide care for elders (Gallagher et al., 1987).

Most investigators have found that the physical health of caregivers does not decline more than the health of persons of similar age and sex who are not caregivers. When compared for mental health, however, caregivers report as many as three times the number of stress-related symptoms as the comparison groups, as well as a decrease in life satisfaction. The more extreme stress-related symptoms can evolve into anxiety and depressive disorders that in turn require professional care. Usually, however, the burden is not so severe and the caregiver bears the burden with little, if any, support from professionals, family, and friends.

The behaviors of debilitated elders that cause serious problems for caregivers often surprise those who are not caregivers. Cleaning up after elders who have an inability to control urination and bowel movements is among the more distasteful of tasks required of caregivers of older adults. Yet Rabins et al. (1982) found that urinary and fetal incontinence were not the most problematic behaviors for families. In a study of the caregivers of fifty-five demented elders, physical violence (75 percent) and memory disturbance (68 percent) were the behaviors of the impaired elder that were the most disturbing to the family. Accusations (50 percent), suspiciousness (48 percent), and striking the caregiver were less frequent complaints. Incontinence was complained of by 62 percent. The stress-related symptom that caregivers cited most commonly were chronic fatigue, anger, depression, family conflict, loss of friends and hobbies with no time for self, and worry that the caregiver would become ill.

ROLE CHANGES

Another problem facing families is the role changes inherent with increased age (Atchley, 1985). The most important role changes to which older persons must adapt are retirement, widowhood, dependency secondary to disability and illness, and change of residence. Though pensions and benefits in retirement are usually available to older adults today, retirement means for the elder that status in the community is lost. Yet the greatest strain that results from retirement may not be the loss of a vocation. Retirement necessitates other changes: that is, the retiree must find a new role. Retired persons are required to become more self-sufficient in negotiating benefits, occupying time, and finding meaningful activities in which to engage. Some marriages are strengthened at retirement whereas others enter a crisis, for a bad marriage may have persisted for many years due to occupations outside the home. Most elders, however, adjust to retirement with little difficulty and find their life more satisfied following retirement.

Widowhood is another role change common to older persons, especially to women (over two-thirds of women over the age of 65 at present are or will become widows). Not only does widowhood deprive the older person of the most intimate and supportive relationship available through most of life, it changes significantly the role of the elder in the community. Social gatherings and events to which couples were invited previously are no longer available to the widow. Widows, especially widowed females, however, tend to form close relations and are quite adept at supporting one another.

Disability and sickness require another role change that, for many elders, is especially disturbing. Dependency is perhaps the most dreaded of role changes. The older person, the patriarch of the family possibly, has been independent financially and physically for over forty years, only to find himself or herself dependent on children. If conflicts existed in the family prior to the need to be dependent (usually due to sickness and disability), these conflicts are usually magnified when the child is forced to take more adult responsibilities (even if the child is middle-aged).

Another role change that is difficult for the elder is a change of residence especially the change to an institution. About 4 percent of the persons over the age of 65 currently reside in institutions. Yet movement from an independent living arrangement that may have been occupied for decades to a retirement community or into the home of the children can be equally disturbing to the elder. Illness, disability, or finances may all contribute to the need for such a move, yet the move itself disrupts social relations and readjusts relations to the family.

When children invite parents into their own homes (or move into the home of the elderly parent), conflicts may arise that undermine the ability of the family to care for an older adult suffering an emotional problem and may even precipitate emotional problems in the elder or other family members (McGreehan and Warburton, 1978). A child who enjoyed his or her own bedroom might be asked to share a room with a sibling to make room for a grandparent. If the grandparent recognizes that he or she has become a source of disruption in the family, then the grandparent may feel guilty, frustrated, and depressed. Grandchildren dislodged from their own rooms may harbor resentment toward the grandparent.

Arguments may arise between parents and children over furnishings of the house. Adult children may wish to furnish their parent's room with new furniture, whereas the parents may wish to bring treasured objects into the adult child's house (including many pieces of furniture). Parents may even ask the adult child to distribute the furniture throughout the child's house.

At times, the elder is expected to perform certain tasks in the family and this can create problems. For sharing the home, retired parents may be expected to babysit grandchildren and great-grandchildren. Elders often resent being "tied down" while their adult children enjoy free time that was not available to the elder during the childrearing years. On the other hand, some elders feel deprived of an important role if they are never asked to care for their grandchildren (as they themselves may have been cared for by their grandparents).

ELDER ABUSE AND NEGLECT

The most severe problem that arises in families of elders suffering emotional or physical problems is elder abuse and neglect. Violence in the home and abuse of family members who are incapable of defending themselves has always existed. In recent years, however, the abuse of elders by their adult children or their spouses has received more media attention. Quinn (1987) listed five ways families abuse their elder members:

1. Physical abuse and neglect may result in bruises, cuts, broken bones, dehydration, and malnutrition.
2. Financial abuse (more common with the elders than physical abuse) results in the older adult's loss of property and possessions because of ill-advised suggestions from family members (usually children) or even fraudulent behavior toward the parents.
3. Violation of basic rights may include not allowing the older adult to vote or open his or her own mail.
4. Psychological abuse usually accompanies these other types of abuses and often consists of threats to abandon the older adult or to place the elder in a nursing home.
5. Self-abuse, such as when the elder refuses to eat or seek medical care for an illness, may stem from the elder's perception that he or she is not loved by the family or it may be the result of an emotional problem.

Evaluating the Family of the Older Adult with Emotional Problems

ESTABLISHING A RELATIONSHIP WITH THE OLDER
ADULT AND THE FAMILY

The evaluation of the family of older adults suffering emotional problems requires skill in assessing the nature of family interactions and skill in facilitating progress through the evaluation (Larson and Blazer, 1984). Following the evaluation of the suffering elder, the professional should evaluate the family alone on at least one occasion. The family session should be held in a room that can comfortably accommodate all relevant members of the patient's family (such as a conference room as opposed to an office). The perception by a family member that there is not enough room for that member thwarts the evaluation process. Attention should initially be directed to the family member who is most influential. Not infrequently in the family of a disturbed elder, an adult child rather than the patient's spouse becomes the spokesperson for the family. Yet the professional must recognize that an isolated conversation with one family member can not only split the professional from the suffering elder but from other family members as well.

Most families protect areas of family stress if they are confronted directly during the initial evaluation. The professional must therefore be gentle in exploring these areas of weakness as they inevitably will be exposed in a family faced with a problem of managing an emotionally disturbed elder.

IDENTIFYING FAMILY ROLES

Once the professional has established a working relationship with the family, he or she should identify members of the family and their roles and characteristics. Physicians often use a genogram to describe the members and the hierarchy of an individual family. By using symbols for males ($\male$) and females ($\female$) and lines to denote relationships between family members, the family as a whole can be pictured. A genogram should indicate members living and dead,

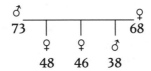

causes of death, ages, separations and/or divorces, illnesses suffered by individual members, and geographic location. With transportation so readily available and virtually all family members a telephone call away, the geographic location is less important today than in previous years. Nevertheless, extreme distances and financial constraints limit the ability of some family members to provide support, especially support in a time of unexpected crisis.

As described above, the development of an emotional problem by an elder places strain upon family roles. Often during a crisis, family members take on specific roles in order to cope adequately and support the elder during the emotional illness. Garetz (1979) described a number of roles that family members may assume when interacting with an elder suffering from an emotional problem. I modified these roles somewhat in a more recent publication (Blazer, 1984).

Facilitator. This individual is a family member who does not want the elder with emotional problems to seek treatment. The facilitator is more comfortable with the way things are, dealing with the dysfunctional elder, and he or she resists any change in this status quo. For example, a facilitator may be more comfortable with an overly dependent and depressed elder than an elder who recovers and asserts his or her independence again. The facilitator presents many obstacles to therapy as he or she attempts to maintain an equilibrium within the family system. In other words, the facilitator believes, either consciously or unconsciously, that the family is better served when the elder remains emotionally disturbed, dependent, and/or dysfunctional.

Victim. This member of the family perceives the emotional problem of the elder as a direct threat. The victim most likely has frequent contact with the elder suffering the emotional problem (and therefore, with professionals who are working with the elder) and may actually criticize professionals for not being able to accomplish anything with the sick elder or seek attention from the professional himself.

Manager. This family member takes charge of the family during a crisis. He or she is calm, organized, and tends to intellectualize contacts with the professional. The manager can be very helpful to the professional in arranging tangible supports but is less able to provide emotional support to the suffering elder or to other family members. Family "managers" often live at some distance from other family members who are more intimately involved in caring for the elder with an emotional problem.

Caregiver. These individuals have an innate need to nurture the elder with emotional problems. Caregivers provide an inexhaustible source of help to severely disabled elders, sometimes maintaining an older adult in the home far beyond the point at which institutionalization is appropriate, as in the case of dementia. Avoiding opportunities for respite, caregivers frequently drive themselves to the point that they cannot perform useful or meaningful activities other than caregiving. When the older person dies, caregivers often suffer a tremendous void, which manifests itself in a severe and prolonged grief reaction. This caregiving activity can be maladaptive when it is motivated by guilt or when it prevents the elder person from achieving greater independence.

Escapee. The escapee withdraws from the family during the crisis of an emotional problem suffered by an elder member and subsequently is blamed for not showing more care and concern for the disturbed elder. The escapee is typically an adult child who has moved some distance from the family. Such individuals often become involved in other altruistic endeavors (religious or civic activities) and therefore may rationalize that they have obligations that prevent devoting time to caring for the elder with emotional problems. Families that experience much interpersonal conflict in times of crises almost always find escapees. Whether consciously or unconsciously, the escapee recognizes the problems within the family and withdraws from the family as a means of self-defense. The escapee may function well outside the family and resist being drawn back into a stressed and conflicted relationship with his or her kin. The family, in turn, displaces its frustration to the escapee.

The elder with the emotional problem. The older person with the problem precipitates the family crisis or has physical and emotional problems that require adaptive changes within the family. Family therapists have recognized for years that the elderly patient (i.e., the presenting problem) in the family may actually be a "ticket" for the family to enter the helping relationship, that is, gives "permission" for the family to talk with the professional about family conflict. The actual problem causing family discord may only be peripherally related to the elder's emotional problem. In other words, the professional may perceive that he or she is asked to treat an elder's emotional problem, whereas the family is seeking help for a most different problem.

These roles (and they may certainly vary from one family to another and all may not be filled in any given family) also change through time. Yet trying to understand the roles of family members and interrelations between those members during the crisis of an elder suffering an emotional problem provides a useful framework for evaluating the elder within the context of the family.

The professional must also evaluate the quantity and quality of interaction within the family (Blazer, 1984). Questions to ask the suffering elder include these:

- How often does your (son, daughter, brother, and so forth) visit you in your home?
- How often do you visit other family members in their homes?
- How often do you contact other family members by phone?
- How many of your family members live within thirty minutes driving distance?
- How often do you visit with your closest friends, either by phone or in person?

EVALUATING FAMILY INTERACTION

The quality of family interaction is more important than the quantity of interaction. Families that are interacting frequently may be so conflicted that they provide little positive and much negative reinforcement to the emotional problems suffered by the older adult. The quality of interaction can be assessed by evaluating the family according to the following parameters (Blazer, 1984).

Compatible vs. conflictual. Do family members usually agree or do they argue over even minor issues? Have old conflicts, especially conflicts between the elder and his or her middle-aged children, been brought to the surface in the midst of a crisis after years of dormancy?

Cohesive vs. fragmented. Does a family remain together in times of crisis? Do family members present their problems as a unit or do they contact professionals individually? An excellent way to determine the cohesiveness of the family is to observe how many persons come with the disturbed elder when a problem presents.

Productive vs. nonproductive. Can the family work together to accomplish the tasks that are necessary to aid the older adult suffering an emotional problem? Has the family demonstrated the ability to work productively in other endeavors, such as in a family business or another crisis? If the older person suffering the emotional problem was reluctant to seek professional help, was the family capable of motivating the elder to undergo a proper evaluation?

Fragile vs. stable. Has the family remained relatively stable, both in its members and interactions, over time? Is the family capable of providing support over an extended period of time? Have marriages within the family been maintained or are divorce and remarriage the norm? Do children and young adults maintain regular contact with their older family members?

Rigid vs. flexible. How fluid are the roles within the family? If the family member who has managed problems in the past becomes incapacitated, dies, or is not available during a crisis, are other members ready and capable of taking the role of manager? Do family members accept changing roles within the family as needed? Are usual family procedures that are mobilized to work through a problem flexible?

The professional must also evaluate the family for their values (Blazer, 1984). What are the family values concerning health? Excellent health is the norm in some families, whereas other families are fraught with both physical and emotional problems. Some families accept illness in an elder (either physical or emotional), whereas others do not tolerate dysfunction. What are the values of the family concerning aging? Do families permit older adults to maintain an active role in the family? Once the elder has retired, whom do family members seek out for support and advice (or even financial assistance)?

The professional must determine the degree to which tangible services can be provided to an older person with an emotional problem by family members. These services could be performed by professionals or family members. How much work and what kind of assistance from outside the family will be necessary to facilitate coping with the emotional problem? For example, to what extent can the family provide transportation for the elder to appointments and social and recreational activities? Can family members administer medications and provide nursing services? Is someone in the family available to supervise the elder (either by checking periodically or by providing continuous supervision)? Is someone available to prepare meals? Can a family member be identified who can undertake, either temporarily or permanently, the task of paying the bills and protecting the legal and financial needs of the elder suffering an emotional problem? If the elder can no longer live alone (yet does not require a nursing home), is there a family member who will provide living quarters?

Finally, the professional should evaluate other stressors that may have an impact on the family (Blazer, 1984). Middle-aged children of an emotionally disturbed elder often are confronting concurrent stressors, such as economic problems (they may have moved to a new home or the children are attending a private college). Since both spouses in mid-life are more likely to be working today than in past years, the availability of children or their spouses to care for the impaired elder has decreased. Another frequent crisis is an emotional problem suffered by an adult child or a grandchild (a mid-life crisis or drug abuse in a grandchild).

Family Interventions

JOINING THE FAMILY

Once the professional has evaluated the emotionally disturbed elder within the context of the family, the professional must "join" the family. Minuchin (1974) suggested that joining the family system occurs when the professional has been accepted as an "honorary family member." Once the professional accepts the family's organizational style, he or she can begin to blend with that style. Families are more reluctant to accept an outsider into the system than the professional is willing to become a part of the family system. A successful professional, however, can provide empathy and understanding of the stress faced by the family and complement family strengths. Statements such as "Sounds as if you have always been a very close family" or "You have always depended on your father and I know it is difficult not to be able to turn to him in this situation" may relax the family and enable members to receive assistance more freely (Larson and Blazer, 1984).

In some situations, the professional may need to take specific responsibilities, such as making decisions that are too painful and difficult for family members. For example, a family may dread making the tough decision of insisting that an older woman be hospitalized for a severe depression, even though they recognize the risk of suicide. A psychiatrist, working effectively with the family, can join the family and take the responsibility for making this decision. The psychiatrist can say, "I know it is difficult to make this decision, but it is a decision that must be made. Let me take the responsibility and you can simply tell your mother that I insisted that she be admitted to the hospital." In such a situation, family members usually ally with the professional, secure that responsibility is not totally placed upon their own shoulders. All too often, however, in our autonomous approach to the treatment of physical and psychiatric disorders, professionals are not able or willing to make such a holistic step as to join the family.

Once necessary decisions during a crisis have been made and the professional understands the structure and functioning of the family, therapeutic goals should be set for family as well as for the elder suffering an emotional problem. These goals include: family therapy (when family problems are contributing to the emotional problems of the elder or when the elder's emotional problem has become too great a burden upon the family); education (such as filling in gaps about the process of aging, the nature of mental and physical disorders, and the realistic expectations of the different therapies); and availability. Following a crisis, reeducation is the most appropriate initial goal. Education should be coordinated, as soon as possible, by garnering resources for the family to meet whatever crises are faced.

FAMILY INTERACTION IN SUSPECTED CASES OF ELDER ABUSE

One of the more difficult tasks facing a professional working with an emotionally disturbed elder is to intervene in cases where abuse is suspected. The best means to prevent elder abuse is through "primary prevention," that is, intervening before abuse has actually occurred but where the risk is recognized. Making known community resources, identifying strains in the family caused by the illness of an elder, and identifying with the angry feelings that can result from another person's emotional disorder are ways in which primary prevention can be practiced. Families and the community should be educated regarding the prevalence of elder abuse and the need to identify the problem early and intervene appropriately. One means by which abuse can be prevented is to encourage the elder and family members to use resources outside the home, such as day care, intermittent hospitalization, and respite care for caregivers. If significant administrative problems have arisen within the family, the suggestion to obtain outside help from either a lawyer or a financial adviser is appropriate.

If conflicts that potentially could lead to abuse are recognized by the professional working with a family, then professional counseling should be made available to enable the family to work through those conflicts and hostile feelings (Steuer and Austin, 1980). In addition to the use of community resources, families can be taught behavioral techniques to handle difficult situations (such as providing a blueprint for working with an elder whose suspicious or hostile behavior encourages retribution from a family member).

Once abuse has occurred, however, a different intervention strategy is necessary—both social and legal. The usual approach to family intervention must be abandoned. Counseling services should be mandatory, though counselors must take a supportive stand toward both the elder and the family. Nevertheless, behaviors bordering on abuse (physical threats) or suggestion of abuse should be strongly censored. At times, even legal resources may be necessary in order to protect an elder from family members. The provision of financial and administrative protection presents a quandary for the professional who cannot become personally involved and must not attempt to form legal judgments.

One of the most important roles of the professional is to enable family members working with emotionally disturbed elders to make contact with and gain strength from the numerous family support programs. Support programs for families of Alzheimer's disease victims, especially the Alzheimer's Disease and Related Diseases Association, are widely available and effective (Gwyther, 1987). Support groups can provide a toll-free telephone number for families to request information and a referral to services relevant for managing a variety of emotional and physical illnesses. Programs also provide peer counseling, gather and catalog specialized information, and provide technical assistance for family members. Support programs also provide an organized advocacy initiative for families suffering the burden of a problem such as Alzheimer's disease. Effective programs require professionals who are facilitators and who encourage program development by volunteers. Once developed, volunteers become the strength and leadership of the program. Nevertheless, continued interaction between professionals and volunteers in such programs is essential for their ongoing success.

Finally, professionals should instruct families about specific ways in which they can reduce the burden of an emotional problem suffered by an elder. A number of guidebooks, such as *The 36-Hour Day* (Mace and Rabins, 1981), are now available for families facing problems with older adults. Despite the importance of family therapy and support, education of the family may be the most important task that the professional undertakes. Most families are capable of providing the best of care for their elder members, if these families possess the necessary information and if they are in touch with the relevant resources.

References

Atchley, R. C. *Social Forces and Aging* (4th ed.). Belmont, CA: Wadsworth, 1985.

Blazer, D. G. "Evaluating the family of the elderly patient." In D. G. Blazer and I. C. Siegler (Eds.), *A Family Approach to Health Care in the Elderly.* Menlo Park, CA: Addison-Wesley Publishing Co., 1984. Pp. 13–31.

Gallagher, D., M. Wrabetz, S. Lovet, S. D. Maestro, and J. Rose. "Depression and other negative affects in family caregivers." In E. Light and B. Liebowitz (Eds.), *Alzheimer's Disease Treatment and Family Stress: Directions for Research.* Washington, DC: U.S. Government Printing Office, 1987. Pp. 218–244.

Garetz, F. K. "Responses of families to health problems in the elderly." Paper presented at the 36th Annual Meeting of the American Geriatric Society, April, 1979.

Gwyther, L. P. "The Duke Aging Center Family Support Program: A grassroots outreach program generates principles and guidelines." *Center Reports on Advances in Research*, 11:1, 1987.

Larson, D., and D. G. Blazer. "Family therapy with the elderly." In D. G. Blazer and I. C. Siegler (Eds.), *A Family Approach to Health Care in the Elderly*. Menlo Park, CA: Addison-Wesley Publishing Co., 1984. Pp. 95–111.

Mace, N. L. and P. V. Rabins. *The 36-Hour Day*. Baltimore: Johns Hopkins, 1981.

McGreehan, D. M., and S. W. Warburton. "How to help families cope with caring for the elderly members." *Geriatrics*, 32:99, 1978.

Miller, K. T., and J. L. Miller. "The family as a system." Paper presented at the Annual Meeting of the American College of Psychiatrists, February, 1979.

Minuchin, S. *Families and Family Therapy*. Cambridge, MA: Harvard University Press, 1974.

Quinn, M. J. "Elder abuse and neglect." In G. L. Maddox (Ed.), *The Encyclopedia of Aging*. New York: Springer Publishing Co., 1987. Pp. 202–204.

Rabins, P. V., N. L. Mace, and M. J. Lucas. "The impact of dementia on the family." *Journal of the American Medical Association*, 248:333, 1982.

Steuer, J., and E. Austin. "Family abuse of the elderly." *Journal of the American Geriatric Society*, 28:372, 1980.

Suggested Reading

Blazer, D. G., and I. C. Siegler (Eds.). *A Family Approach to Health Care in the Elderly*. Menlo Park, CA: Addison-Wesley Publishing Co., 1984.

Bumagin, V. E., and K. F. Hirn. *Helping the Aging Family*. Glenview, IL: Scott, Foresman and Co., 1990.

Maddox, G. L. (Ed.). *The Encyclopedia of Aging*. New York: Springer Publishing Company, 1987.

Silverstone, B., and A. Burack-Weiss. *Social Work Practice with the Frail Elderly and their Families*. Springfield, IL: Charles C. Thomas, 1983.

Tilson, D. (Ed.). *Aging in Place: Supporting the Frail Elderly in Residential Environments*. Glenview, IL: Scott, Foresman and Co., 1990.

Troll, L., S. J. Miller, and R. C. Atchley. *Families in Later Life*. Belmont, CA: Wadsworth, 1979.

CHAPTER THIRTEEN

Successful Aging

As discussed in Chapter 1, successful aging cannot be so simply defined as the absence of physical and emotional problems faced by the elderly. Indeed, some characteristics of aging can be modified. Rowe and Kahn (1987) suggest that the effects of the aging process have been exaggerated, and the potential for modifying this process by diet, exercise, change in personal habits, and social engagement is underestimated. They suggest that our concepts of aging should be adjusted so that we do not view extrinsic factors as simply facilitating the losses of aging. Rather, these factors can play a neutral or even a positive role. The extreme variability at any age of physical, psychological, and social function substantiates this view. In other words, differences across the life cycle are not much more varied than differences across a sample of older adults at a given age.

The professional plays an important part in the elder's aging process. Through intervention, a professional can aid both the depressed elder, who needs help in recovering from a major depression, and the demoralized elder, who does not suffer major depression or dysthymia but suffers nevertheless. These interventions help promote successful later years for elders, and these years can become the happiest period of an individual's life.

The following is an example of a successfully aging elder.

The old professor had retired from the university ten years ago. At his retirement at age 65, he was known as "the old professor." The junior faculty had known him only by name and reputation. He contributed textbooks and research reports to his field of study; he had a reputation as an excellent teacher (many faculty from other departments had studied with him as undergraduates); and he had acted as a consultant to other universities throughout the country. Today he was returning to his university at the request of the department chairman, who had invited him to teach a course during the fall semester.

Though he was not up on the latest findings in his field, those who talked with the old professor in the faculty lounge did appreciate his understanding of the field and the philosophical orientation he brought to their own investigative efforts. When a young faculty member described her research, the old professor asked her many detailed questions about her methods, why she had formulated the hypotheses as she had, and what she expected to conclude. Though he was not as diligent in reading the journals as previously, the old professor maintained a curiosity about developments in the field. During the semester, he attended many lectures given by the current faculty. Often, at the conclusion of the lecture, he would be the first to approach the professor to ask a question about the presentation.

During the semester, the faculty became more curious about the old professor as well. What had he done for the ten years since retirement? Though he had visited the campus occasionally, the new faculty had not talked with him, for he had never remained long enough to maintain a conversation.

The senior faculty who had known the old professor prior to his retirement were not surprised to learn that he continued an active consulting practice. Twenty to thirty times a year, the old professor would speak to a symposium, participate in a workshop, or consult with a fledgling department in another state. Two to three times per year, he traveled abroad for similar activities. As his consulting practice through the years had provided an ample income in addition to his retirement benefits from the university, he traveled often with his wife (who had also taught in the university). They enjoyed driving to the sights of symposia he presented, for previously he had little time and was forced to take airplanes. Usually, they would remain two or three days visiting friends, touring, and relaxing.

When not consulting, the old professor and his wife enjoyed their mountain cottage, an investment made for enjoyment in retirement and as a financial shelter some thirty years previously. His wife, who had taught in the department of botany, continued her lifelong interest in the flora of the Appalachian Mountains. As he was not interested in flowers, the old professor enjoyed the golf courses (he usually played eighteen holes three to four days every week while they were in the mountains). Otherwise, he enjoyed reading the books and the magazines that he had never been able to read before. His reading had drifted from the technical articles of his specialty into more philosophical and historical works regarding his field. He jokingly (perhaps not entirely) said that he planned to write a final book placing his field of study in some historical and philosophical context. The senior faculty who knew his work had often commented on his relaxed and philosophical view of his field. They had appreciated him in years past for placing changes in the field, as well as crises in university life, into perspective. As far back as they could remember, he had been a stabilizing force in a stormy environment.

Junior faculty in the department were especially surprised at his physical activity. The old professor walked two miles to the campus each day from his home and returned each night. He continued to play golf at least once a week while teaching and attending classes. They were surprised to hear that he scored "in the mid 80s," a level of performance that was no worse than when he played regularly at the age of 45. The old professor did complain of a few "aches and pains" but said that these rarely slowed him down. He noticed a little problem with his memory, but not for anything that he valued. He had never been hospitalized, for, "Thank the good Lord, I had the wisdom to choose parents who were healthy and lived into their nineties." His mother had lived to the age of 95 and his father to 97. Both remained in excellent health until their deaths two and three years prior to his return to campus.

As the semester neared an end, a young assistant professor asked the old professor his secret for aging so gracefully. After a pithy comment challenging the suggestion that he was "aged," the old professor suggested a few guiding principles. For example, he had always attempted to live his life in moderation, never smoking and limiting his alcohol consumption to one or two glasses of wine a day. Always a curious person, he had looked forward to retirement and had planned a course of reading for twenty years beginning at age 65. He currently was halfway through this reading program. He had been most careful with his money and was thankful that he and his wife possessed the financial resources to do as they wished. He also launched into a short diatribe about "old values" which the young professor did not particularly care to hear.

When spring semester arrived and the old professor was no longer around, the young assistant professor reflected upon his observation and conversations with the old professor. Sometimes, the old professor had irritated him, for he did not appear to be as informed as he should for the responsibilities of teaching at the university. He believed the old professor philosophized too much and neglected the data. In addition, he realized that he himself would never share a value orientation with the old professor. Nevertheless, he admired the professor for his contribution to the field over many years and hoped that his retirement would be as successful as that of his elderly colleague. When he attempted to review what he knew about the older professor, looking for guidelines to successful aging, he was disappointed that he could garner so few generalizations from the experience.

The Concept of Successful Aging

VITALITY

As the younger professor discovered, there is no specific formula for successful aging, although there are certain traits that successfully aging elders seem to possess. One of these is *vitality*. In their provocative book *Vitality and Aging*, Fries and Crapo (1981) note that although the limits of the life span of homo sapiens has not increased for hundreds of years (theorized to range between 90 and 110 years), the age of people who approach the limits of the life span has increased dramatically. Not only are people living longer, they are healthier as they enter and progress through what is commonly considered "late life." In other words, there is a new vitality among older adults in late life, as Robert Browning wrote in "Rabbi Ben Ezra":

Grow old along with me!
The best is yet to be,
The last of life, for which the first was made. . .

As the underlying cause of death for many elders is a decrease in the defense mechanisms of the organism due to senescence (or primary aging), the prevention and effective treatment of diseases will extend life-long vitality and decrease the chronicity of disease. Many investigators have taken issue with Fries and Crapo, reporting that the increased life expectancy of elders in the United States is actually accompanied by an increase in years of chronicity. Nevertheless, the goal of a society of elders less plagued by chronic illnesses and treated more effectively for these illnesses—that is, a more vigorous society of elders—is within our grasp.

RESILIENCE

Yet another concept associated with the successfully aging elder is *resilience*. The older adult who ages successfully is the older adult who can adapt successfully to a variety of expected and unexpected physical, psychological, and social stressors. Resilience from the biologic perspective may derive from good physical health and functioning. For example, the older woman who has never smoked, has carefully controlled her weight, and has participated in aerobic exercises adapts much better to the physical stressor of pneumonia than the woman who has smoked, has not exercised, and is obese. The older man who has developed a variety of interests and social relations throughout his adult life and has maintained these into retirement is usually more capable of adapting to the loss of his spouse than the man who has few interests and has been socially dependent on his wife through the retirement years.

Resilience may be biologically innate and variable across individuals. For example, some persons adjust much more easily than others to rapid changes in time zones (that is, they adjust to jet lag better than others). For the most part, however, resilience is modifiable throughout the life cycle.

ADAPTIVE ABILITY

Closely associated with the concept of resilience is the concept of *adaptation*. Aging, indeed life itself, is characterized by confronting and adapting to biologic, psychological, and social challenges. Positive adaptation is reflected in satisfaction with the quality of life among persons in late life (Butt and Beiser, 1987). According to Butt and Beiser, adaptation across the life span can be conceived by two different models. The first is the cognitive appraisal model of Lazarus (1966), which focuses upon how well the individual copes with stressful situations. Successful aging can be operationalized as the ability of the elder to adapt to stressors. The second is the subjective well-being model (Campbell et al., 1976), which focuses upon the individual satisfaction with personal and social resources and experiences. Successful aging can therefore be operationalized as satisfaction of individuals across a number of life domains, such as the satisfaction with job relations, human relations, material needs, and religion.

AUTONOMY AND CONTROL

Rodin (1986) has emphasized the importance of maintaining *autonomy and control* for successful aging. To the extent that individuals can make decisions about their activities, the nature of their participation in these activities, the sequencing of activities, and the pace of activities, they adapt successfully. Not only are elders more discouraged and less satisfied with their lives when they perceive themselves out of control, they perform less well and may be at increased risk for physical illness or injury. A study by Krantz and Schulz (1980) illustrates the importance of autonomy. These investigators conducted an experiment in which patients who were scheduled to be admitted to a nursing home were divided into groups. Some of these individuals were given a choice as to when they would move into a nursing home, a choice of the nursing home into which they moved, and choices regarding arrangements after the move. In contrast to subjects not given these choices, who experienced a number of negative changes in their health after admission into a nursing home, the elders given some choices suffered little decline in health from the move and no change in life satisfaction.

INTEGRITY

Erik Erikson (1987) recently expanded his theory that *integrity* is a necessity for successful aging. In Erikson's epigenetic theory of development, he emphasized the dynamic balance of opposites at each of the eight stages of life. For example, the infant struggles to develop basic trust and overcome basic mistrust. In Erikson's theory, each stage contributes to a successful adaptation to succeeding stages. Successful transition from infancy leads to the characteristic of hope in the individual. The last of Erikson's stages is called "integrity vs. despair." The task of the elder is to reflect on his or her life, catalog and review experiences and accomplishments, and integrate these memories into a meaning of one's life. Failure to accomplish integration leads to despair. Successful integration leads to wisdom: "The sense of "I," in old age, still has a once-for-all chance of transcending time-bound identities and sensing, if only in the simplest terms, an all-human and existential identity like that which the world religions and ideologies have attempted to create . . ." (Erikson et al., 1987).

WISDOM

Erikson and his colleagues, in their emphasis on integrity, provide the bridge to yet another concept associated with successful aging—wisdom. According to Erikson, wisdom is detached concern with life itself in the face of death. Wisdom not only persists, it conveys the integrity of experience to others, despite the decline of physical and mental functions. Wisdom, like successful aging, is more difficult to define than to illustrate. For example, Smith et al. (1985) suggest two general and three specific criteria essential for "wise" judgment:

1. Good judgment, good advice and/or insightful commentary
2. Rich (or good), factual, and procedural knowledge in the domain in terms of depth and scope
3. Extensive contextualism (the person/issue in detailed background)
4. Extensive relativism (person/issue in dialectic setting of different values and contending ideas)
5. Extensive uncertainty (articulation of unpredictable, changeable elements)

SOCIAL INTEGRATION

Successful aging can also be conceived in terms of *social integration*. Maddox (1987) cites the work of Lawton et al. (1973), which focused upon a tradition of persons/context fitting. Individuals can be matched or mismatched in terms of their own capabilities and the contextual opportunities available to them. Yet integration not only depends on the fitting of the individual to social context and institutions, these very institutions may need to be adapted to the older adult. For example, the difficulties older persons experience in obtaining adequate medical services were greatly decreased with the advent of Medicare. Though this national insurance policy has been plagued with many difficulties, there is little doubt that older adults in the latter twentieth century have benefitted greatly from uniform access to health care. As the economic well-being of elders improves, however, the system must be modified to place less strain on society and transfer some additional financial responsibilities to the elderly population. To the extent that our society can adapt to the older adult and his or her needs and elders can adapt to the needs of society, elders will be better integrated into our society. Social integration not only facilitates the physical, psychological, and social well-being of elders, it also benefits society by releasing the energies and talents of elders that can be used by our society.

Interventions That Promote Successful Aging

A biopsychosocial approach to emotional problems experienced by elders is the best means by which coping with those problems can be facilitated. Many so-called processes of aging are modifiable. Elders can change behaviors to slow secondary aging and prevent diseases related to aging. Fries and Crapo (1981) suggest many changes in health practices that can increase biologic vitality in late life. A physically healthy elder is an elder who suffers less from emotional problems. Persons who exercise regularly and who are disciplined enough to control their diet, quit smoking, and so on, are also less likely to suffer many emotional problems (especially problems with depression and anxiety). Certainly the impact of an emotional problem in late life that undermines motivation and concentration, such as a severe biologic depression, can interrupt the practice of good health habits. Nevertheless, the practice of good health habits is one means to improve the physical and emotional well-being of the elder.

IMPROVED HEALTH HABITS

What are the habits that can be modified and what is the expected result? Cessation of smoking and weight loss improve cardiac reserve, increase physical endurance, increase pulmonary reserve, decrease serum cholesterol (a risk factor for heart attacks), and lower blood pressure. Proper care of teeth and gums through dieting reduces dental decay, postpones the necessity for false teeth, and maintains the ability of the elder to eat a variety of foods. Avoiding exposure to the sun decreases the likelihood of age-related skin problems, especially skin cancer (as was suffered by former President Reagan) and wrinkling of the skin. Salt limitation (along with weight control) reduces blood pressure. A diet high in protein and low in carbohydrates improves "glucose tolerance," which in turn decreases the risk for diabetes. Even when health habits are changed late in life (for example, in the late seventies or early eighties), these changes contribute to a more vigorous and possibly extended life.

EXERCISE

Exercise is an excellent means to improve physiologic well-being and promote successful aging. Persons over the age of 60 decrease their activities dramatically. Blumenthal and Williams (1982) reviewed the evidence that suggests exercise reverses the adverse physical and psychological changes that accompany aging. The present cohort of older adults, however, is much less likely to participate in vigorous exercise. In a Canadian survey, more than 8 percent of persons 25 to 64 years old participated in some sport three or more hours per week and another 5 percent participated in some vigorous activity. Only 3 percent of persons 65 to 69 participated in such sports and 3 percent participated in other activities. The elderly were the least likely, in a survey conducted by the Harris poll, to predict that they would become involved in some exercise program in the future.

Nevertheless, a number of programs have been developed that are "user friendly" to older adults and encourage them to participate in exercise. For example, the Duke University Preventive Approach to Cardiology (DUPAC) program is targeted for persons in mid-life and late life. Participants meet each morning, and program instructors emphasize exercise, conditioning, diet modification, and stress management as a strategy for health maintenance and reha-bilitation from cardiac illness. The trained personnel work with the older participants to develop and pace an individualized exercise program and, in case of an emergency, are certified in cardiopulmonary resuscitation and other forms of medical assistance. Though most of these older persons cannot jog initially and tire within a short time with vigorous walking, by the end of the program virtually all participants are doing at least some aerobic exercises. The program lasts for ten weeks.

Blumenthal and Williams (1982) demonstrated that the program was associated not only with improved physical conditioning but also improvement in the psychologic condition of older participants. They found that both state and trait anxiety of participants decreased after the ten-week program. (State anxiety is how the person feels "now" and trait anxiety is how the person generally feels.)

SECONDARY PREVENTION

Another approach to successful aging derives from the public health concept of secondary prevention. Preventive health care is not just preventing the onset of an illness (i.e., primary prevention). Once an illness has been detected, such as coronary heart disease, early intervention (through diet, weight loss, and careful exercise) can reduce the likelihood that the illness will progress. Secondary prevention is not only applicable to the physical problems. If an older adult begins to feel lonely, isolated, or "bored," he or she should not wait until these lonely, depressed feelings multiply into a full-fledged episode of depression. Rather, the elder should seek intervention when the symptoms first appear. Such secondary prevention is much more effective than tertiary prevention, that is, the chronic and prolonged rehabilitation process that occurs after an illness, emotional or physical, has expressed itself fully.

LIFELONG LEARNING

Another intervention to promote successful aging is a commitment to lifelong learning. Adult education has become increasingly prevalent in the United States, and the education of older people has developed primarily from the adult education movement (Peterson, 1987). We in the United States and other Western countries live in a society that values learning. Skills and knowledge required in early years of training, whether in automotive mechanics, law, or medicine, must be updated to accommodate the expansion of knowledge and the acquisition of new skills required to prosper and survive. Many programs have arisen to accommodate the need for continued education, including night courses at community colleges and public schools, special university programs (such as nightly classes in order to obtain a master's degree), special programs at libraries and museums, educational activities at clubs, and continuing education programs within corporations.

Most gerontologists today recognize that the education of the older adult is not focused exclusively on instructions that assist in dealing with the difficulties and crises of old age (such as preretirement planning). Rather, elders have an ability to grow and develop throughout their latter years as they did through their early years.

One of the more popular continuing education activities among the elderly is the Elderhostel program, which includes education in the arts and the humanities as well as nature programs. This program is especially relevant to persons sixty and older, for the subject matter and style of instruction is not focused on acquiring new facts and specific skills to increase productivity, but rather on broadening the interest and knowledge of individuals. Education in the arts and humanities assists elders in integrating their lives and the course of history during their lives more effectively. Older persons in such programs have pursued various arts, such as painting, ceramics, theater, photography, and even dance. Many elders write, perhaps fiction, poetry, history, or an autobiography. The translation of oral history they have inherited into books, plays, or other permanent records has been of interest to elders in recent years (Moody, 1987). Western society is therefore following the course of Eastern cultures, such as India, China, and Japan, in which old age is viewed as an appropriate time for spiritual exploration and artistic development. Those who believe that late life is a time to "disengage" from social interaction suggest that social activities be replaced with opportunities for such personal growth and creativity.

ACTIVITY

Others, however, have challenged the so-called disengagement theory of aging. Cumming and Henry (1961), possibly following the age-old wisdom of Eastern cultures, suggested that nature had programmed elders to achieve life satisfaction in late life by separating themselves from their social involvements and turning their interests and energies inward. Much debate followed this theory of successful aging. Maddox (1987) challenged this theory, suggesting that elders can age successfully by taking a variety of paths. One path is the maintenance of previous activities, that is, the "activity theory" (Havighurst and Albrecht, 1953). These investigators postulated that individuals should maintain high levels of activity in late life in order to sustain their psychological and social well-being. Inactivity, rather than leading to life satisfaction, frequently leads to deterioration and illness. The successfully aging elder may pursue a number of interests during this successful aging and one must not assume that relaxation, social withdrawal, and contemplation are the preferred norm for the end of the life cycle.

Successful aging can be pursued along a variety of paths. Most older persons are reported to be healthy and independent. Each of us who have devoted our lives to the care of older adults suffering emotional problems must not be so short-sighted as to be satisfied merely with relieving that problem. We must recognize the potential of the elder to modify his or her own life, not only to increase the potential for adaptation and resiliency but also to improve life satisfaction and bring meaning to life in the later years.

References

Blumenthal, J. A., and R. S. Williams. "Exercise and aging: The use of physical health in health enhancement." *Center Reports on Advances in Research* 6:1, 1982.

Butt, D. S., and M. Beiser. "Successful aging: A theme for international psychology." *Psychology and Aging*, 2:87, 1987.

Campbell, A., P. Converse, and W. Rogers. *The Quality of American Life*. New York: Russell Sage Foundation, 1976.

Cumming, E., and W. Henry. *Growing Old: The Process of Disengagement*. New York: Basic Books, 1961.

Erickson, E. H., J. M. Erickson, and H. Q. Kibnick. *Vital Involvement in Old Age*. New York: W. W. Norton, 1987.

Fries, J. F., and L. M. Crapo. *Vitality and Aging: Implications of the Rectangular Curve*. San Francisco: W. H. Freeman and Co., 1981.

Havighurst, R. J., and R. Albrecht. *Older People*. New York: Longmans Green, 1953.

Krantz, D., and R. Schulz. "Personal control and health: Some applications to crises of middle and old age." In A. Buam and J. Singer (Eds.), *Advances in Environmental Psychology*. Hilldale, NJ: Erlbaum, 1980. Pp. 23–57.

Lawton, P., and L. Nahemow. "Ecology and the aging process." In C. Eistorfer and P. Lawton (Eds.), *Adult Development in Aging*. Washington, DC: American Psychological Association, 1973. Pp. 55–79.

Lazarus, R. S. *Psychological Stress and the Coping Process*. New York: McGraw-Hill, 1966.

Maddox, G. L. "Aging and well-being." Boettner Lecture, Bryn Mawr, PA. 1987.

Moody, H. R. "Humanities and the arts." In G. L. Maddox (Ed.), *The Encyclopedia of Aging*. New York: Springer Publishing Co., 1987. Pp. 338–340.

Peterson, D. A. "Adult education." In G. L. Maddox (Ed.), *The Encyclopedia of Aging*. New York: Springer Publishing Co., 1987. Pp. 9–10.

Rodin, J. "Control and well being in the elderly." *Science*, 233:1271, 1986.

Rowe, J. W., and R. L. Kahn. "Human aging: Usual and successful." *Science*, 237:143, 1987.

Smith, J. R. A. Dixon, and P. B. Baltes. "Expertise and right planning: A new research approach to investigating aspects to wisdom." Unpublished manuscript. Berlin, FRG: Max Planck Institute for Human Development and Education, 1985.

Suggested Reading

Comfort, A. *A Good Age*. New York: Crown Publishing, 1976.

Downs, H., and R. J. Roll. *The Best Years Book*. New York: Delacorte Press/Eleanor Friede, 1981.

Erikson, E., J. M. Erikson, and H. Q. Kibnick. *Vital Involvement in Old Age*. New York: W. W. Norton, 1987.

Lyell, R. G. (Ed.). *Middle Age, Old Age: Short Stories, Poems, Plays, and Essays on Aging*. New York: Harcourt Brace Jovanovich, 1980.

McKee, P., and H. Kauppinen. *The Art of Aging: A Celebration of Old Age in Western Art*. New York: Human Sciences Press, 1987.

Index